# A Life to Rescue:

## The True Story of a Child Freed from the Bonds of Autism

Written by
Karen Michelle Graham

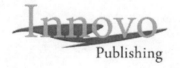

Publishing

Published by
Innovo Publishing, LLC
www.innovopublishing.com
1-888-546-2111

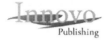
Publishing

Providing Full-Service Publishing Services for
Christian Organizations & Authors: Hardbacks, Paperbacks,
eBooks, Audio Books, & iPhone/iPad Books

**A LIFE TO RESCUE:**
**The True Story of a Child Freed from the Bonds of Autism**
Copyright © 2010 by Karen Michelle Graham
All rights reserved.

ISBN 13: 978-1-936076-25-3
ISBN 10: 1-936076-25-X

Cover Design & Interior Layout: Innovo Publishing, LLC

Printed in the United States of America
U.S. Printing History

First Edition: May 2010

This book is dedicated to

My son Jeremy

and to the autism community—parents, professionals,
and children and adults with autism

Karen Michelle Graham is a pseudonym, used to protect her son's privacy.

Most of the names in this book have been changed. Actual first names were used in the case of the therapists except where noted.

Real names have been used in the following cases: Dr. Ivar Lovaas, Dr. Kotsanis, Dr. Susan Nichol, Dr. Daniel, Dr. Roy Luepnitz, Crystal Burns, Kristie Ramseier, and Dr. Greenspan.

# Acknowledgments

Many heartfelt thanks to:

My husband Randall—his love, support, and hard work blesses my life every day.

My daughter Jennifer—her undying love for her brother and the sacrifices she made for his sake.

Our therapists (Jeremy's heroes), Heather, Heidi, Zach, Jessica, Stephanie, Jill, Vicki, Megan, and all the other dear ones who came in and out of our home. Each one blessed our lives. Thank you for helping us rescue Jeremy from autism.

My friends Kelly and Natalie and all the moms who contributed moral support and brought their children for playtime.

Our consultants, Crystal Burns Held and Kristie Ramseier.

My sisters Rebecca, Mary, Liz, and Ann—their love and prayers helped carry the load. Thanks for listening to me for hours on end.

My sister Ann—thank you for your financial contribution to therapy.

My sister-in-law Paula—thank you for the video camera to record workshops.

My writing friends Donna, Marilyn, Marge, Ike, Carol, and Chris—for your advice and suggestions on the writing of this book.

The Wisconsin Early Autism Project and Dr. Glen Sallows.

If I missed anyone, please know that I appreciate every word of encouragement and every prayer that was given during our crisis.

# Table of Contents

# CHAPTER ONE:
# STOP THE EARTH'S ROTATION—
# I WANT TO GET OFF

**S**ummer 1994

For a romantic like me, life had been ideal. Randall, my husband of fifteen years, was my hero, and we had two beautiful children.

But in the past months, things had changed. Something was terribly wrong with my two-year-old son Jeremy. I bit my lower lip as I sat in the waiting room at our pediatric clinic thinking about the questions I would ask his doctor. First, what was normal behavior for a two-year-old child? Jeremy's behavior didn't match my idea of the terrible twos. And when would he start talking? The childrearing manuals didn't cover what we were going through.

I needed answers.

Jeremy moved to a nearby play table while Jennifer, my six-year-old, sat obediently next to me. Children and parents milled in and out of the large clinic. I glanced at the aquarium and noticed a couple of children observing the fish. Why had Jeremy never wanted to look at the fish?

Tapping Jeremy's arm, I pointed to the aquarium. "Jeremy, look at the fish."

Jeremy spun the beads on a toy mounted on a play table. The red, blue, and yellow maze with colorful beads captured his attention. I frowned. Why the beads and nothing else?

Frustrated and mystified, I sat back down and stared at him. Cute. Blond. Healthy-looking. He was losing his baby fat and thinning out, growing tall for his age. I sighed. He was such a sweetie. With that thought, uncertainty flowed over me. Sweet was the only character trait I could come up with to describe him. I should be able to make a long list of characteristics. Where was his personality? Watching Jennifer and other children, I knew I could describe one as bossy and talkative or another as silly and mischievous, but Jeremy was merely sweet.

A nurse walked from the hallway into the waiting area. "Jeremy Graham."

I stood and walked over to get Jeremy, balancing his diaper bag on my shoulder. Jennifer followed behind us.

In a few minutes, the nurse lifted Jeremy and placed him on the scales. He had other ideas. Crying and fighting the nurse, he flung himself to the floor, progressing into a full-fledged tantrum. What was the matter? It didn't hurt to get weighed. Jennifer stepped to the side to get out of his way. I didn't blame her.

A struggle ensued while I lifted him off the floor and tried reasoning with him.

By the time we saw the doctor, frustration had shattered my patience. I felt everyone within hearing range must be experiencing the same irritation. Once in the examination room, I didn't waste time. "Dr. Nickel, shouldn't Jeremy be talking?"

Dr. Susan Nickel looked past me to care for Jeremy. "I wouldn't worry about it. A lot of two-year-old boys aren't talking yet."

I sighed.

"But he's lost words. When he was twelve months old, he had about ten words. He used to say *dog, toy, mine, more, no,* and *mom.* He has lost all those words. Now all I get is the 'm' sound for everything."

Dr. Nickel frowned. "Hi, Jeremy."

Jeremy stared blankly ahead of him.

The doctor made silly sounds and faces.

Still no response. Why didn't he laugh at her? He wasn't sick. "Jeremy, look at this." She handed Jeremy her stethoscope and turned it in his hand. Despite her gentle, slow pace, he gazed past her as if she wasn't there.

Jeremy didn't show any curiosity regarding the stethoscope. I would expect a child his age to show more interest. She stuck a small pointed medical flashlight into one of his ears to check it. He cried and fought, flinging his arms and struggling to get off the examination table. Jennifer stared wide-eyed.

"Just a moment. I need to get some help." Dr. Nickel left and returned with a male nurse who held Jeremy down for the rest of the examination.

*I can't understand this. Jennifer never reacted like this. All kids are different,* I tried to reassure myself. *He'll outgrow his tantrums.*

The doctor finished checking Jeremy's ears and turned to me. "I really would like a child development specialist to see Jeremy. I'll give you a referral, and let's see what she says."

Dr. Nickel followed us out to the waiting room. While I took care of the paperwork, she continued trying to get Jeremy's attention.

"Jeremy, look at the fish!" I didn't bother telling her I had tried this before without success. Dr. Nickel peeked over at him and pointed to the fish aquarium. But Jeremy walked over and whirled the beads, once again.

Glancing at my watch, I realized Dr. Nickel had spent forty minutes instead of the typical ten minutes with Jeremy. She was booked solid most of the time. What could this mean?

Driving home, the questions and frustration grew like weeds. What's wrong? Glancing back at Jeremy through the rearview mirror, I prayed, *Lord, please help. I don't understand what's going on with my son.*

11

A few days later, while Jennifer was in school, I buckled Jeremy into his car seat and drove to the grocery store. At the stop sign, I turned and looked at him as he stared out the window. "Jeremy, do you want a cracker?" I waited for my answer.

Silence. He didn't even look at me. Frantic to get some language out of him, I raised my voice like one would speak to a deaf person. "Did you hear me? Do you want a cracker? Yes or no?"

"Yes or no," Jeremy echoed. This rare language from him merely echoed my speech. He stared out the window. His behavior came across as just plain odd. A numbing pain settled in my heart. I didn't understand him.

*Maybe he has Attention Deficit Disorder. No, not my beautiful, precious boy.* Peeking quickly in the rearview mirror, I looked at Jeremy with his blond hair curled around the back of his neck and his blue eyes that looked out from long eyelashes. Strangers often commented on his extraordinary eyes. When he was one year old, a daycare worker had called him a heartbreaker.

*God, what's wrong with Jeremy?*

I asked my mother, my sisters, and my friends the same question, but no one had an answer until one evening, some friends had come to visit, and I started telling my friend, Andrea, my worries. "Jeremy stares into space a lot and doesn't respond to his name. Something's not right."

Andrea frowned. "That sounds like my brother, Jim. When he was small, he could stare for hours at the water sprinkler."

"Jeremy's not that bad." I had heard about Jim and had a vague idea about his problems, but I didn't ask what his disability was. I'm not sure why, whether it was out of politeness or some sort of subconscious denial. "Well, I'm going to have his hearing checked."

Some days later, Jeremy and I sat in the ear specialist's office, waiting for the result of his hearing test.

"His hearing is fine," the ear specialist said. "Why do you suspect deafness?"

"Because when I call his name, he doesn't answer me. I usually raise my voice so I can get his attention."

"Don't do that. He can hear you."

\*\*\*

At the breakfast table the next morning, I looked across at my husband while he read the morning newspaper. "Randall, I don't think I should leave Jeremy and go to work."

"He'll be fine. The babysitter will do a great job." Randall took a bite of oatmeal and set the newspaper aside.

"Is it worth the hour and fifteen minute drive one way to Austin just to work only..." I stopped and pushed my fingers through my hair. I had quit my full time job to spend more time with Jeremy but had returned two days a week as a contract employee. "I've put a lot into my career, but let someone else program their computer. Jeremy needs me."

"I understand, honey, but you need to fulfill your commitment on this contract job."

"You're right. I guess the money won't hurt us either." I smiled, but I didn't feel convinced. "I'll see you this afternoon. Tell the babysitter not to let Jeremy watch too much TV, okay?"

I stood up, kissed him, and left, leaving him to wake the kids and greet the babysitter.

As I made the familiar drive south on I-35 to Austin, I planned my schedule. Jeremy's appointment with the child development specialist would be next week. Thoughts of his appointment brought to the surface my worries for Jeremy. Concern for him seldom left me. Had I done something wrong to cause Jeremy to be unresponsive?

Worrying was getting me nowhere. I forced myself to think about the responsibilities at work and made a mental to-do list for the workday. Abruptly, a thought broke through my brainstorming like a news flash.

*What's wrong with Jeremy happened in the womb!* A voice from within me said.

Could this be God speaking to me? I'd been blaming myself for weeks for Jeremy's problems and asking God questions.

*Lord, it wasn't the awful daycare I put Jeremy in when he was a baby, was it? Or the time the daycare worker spilled bleach on him and left him like that? Could that cause brain damage?*

My mind searched for something I could have done to cause Jeremy's problems. I exhaled slowly to relieve the tension. Maybe there were problems during my pregnancy that I was unaware of. *Lord, you know how careful I was with my health when I was pregnant with Jeremy. I did the best I could. I'm not going to feel guilty anymore, Lord. This is not my fault.*

The realization that I wasn't to blame settled over me, giving me comfort and eliminating the question of my possible guilt forever. I felt God's mercy surround me. He cared.

\*\*\*

About a week after this experience, I continued the search for answers to Jeremy's problems. I prayed as I got him ready for the visit to the child development specialist. *Lord, please help the doctor understand what's going on with Jeremy. Even if it's bad, I need to know.* With Jennifer at school, I was freed up to give Jeremy my full attention. I grabbed the diaper bag, buckled Jeremy into his car seat, and left for the appointment.

Later, in an examination room waiting for the doctor, I watched Jeremy play with a toy elephant, the prayer still fresh on my lips. Tension caused my neck to ache. I made an effort to relax.

Finally, the door opened, and a petite, fifty-something woman walked into the room and introduced herself as Dr. Daniel.

After my own introduction, I turned and looked at Jeremy as he picked up a toy car. Then I addressed the doctor. "I'm worried about my son. He's not talking and seems to have lost words." I continued my list of concerns, giving her the examples of him echoing "yes or no," and the fact that he did not respond to his name.

A LIFE TO RESCUE

Dr. Daniel asked me a few questions, observed Jeremy, and tried unsuccessfully to get him to interact with her. Then she hesitated, excused herself, and returned shortly with a booklet and papers.

Before the words came out of her mouth, I knew trouble loomed in the future for my family.

"I believe Jeremy has one of these problems," she said. She handed me material on autism and PDD (pervasive developmental disorder). "He is probably autistic or maybe it's PDD. You will know which one when you read the material. The diagnosis is based on his behaviors, so you will know better than I do. Just observe him."

Was this all she was going to say? I blinked and stared at her, waiting expectantly, but she opened the door and gave me instructions on when to make the next appointment. Then she left.

I knew almost nothing about autism, and I had never heard of PDD.

A dull pain settled in my chest. It felt like the doctor was a messenger from the War Department assigned to inform the families of dead and missing loved ones. Numbly, I switched to autopilot, picked up the diaper bag, and checked out at the reception desk. I hurried away in a cloud of pain. I wanted to be alone to figure this out.

Later, I found out that autism and PDD are diagnosed from a list of 16 diagnostic criteria falling in three major categories—verbal impairment, nonverbal communication, and social impairment. Autism is diagnosed when the child shows eight of the 16 symptoms and a minimum number in each category. Others will fall into the PDD if less than eight (Gerlach, 1996).

\*\*\*

I arrived home to an empty house and set Jeremy in the playroom with his plastic animals. Then I opened the booklets. Words like *grim, incapacitating, life-long* and *incurable* poured from the literature on autism. The material described children who could not speak. Some spent their time lining up objects or flapping

15

their hands. Though I knew little about the disability, hopelessness hit me with the certainty of the news. Wave after wave of discouragement and grief struck me.

My baby! All the hopes and dreams my husband and I had for our son's future swept away in one powerful blow. Tears flowed down my face. Someone might as well have given me a death sentence for my two-year-old son. This could not be happening. I prayed, but found no comfort. Each word in the brochures felt like a physical blow to my chest.

Then I analyzed the behaviors listed in the booklet, *An Introduction to Your Child Who Has Autism* (Centerwall, 1989).

Common Autistic Behaviors: 1. No cuddling. *He only allows me to cuddle him and no one else. I wonder if that counts.*

2. Resistance to change in routine. *Yes, he is resistant to change. When we moved to another house, he held on to my neck with a death grip at bedtime because of the unfamiliar surroundings.*

3. No eye contact. *This is one of his worst problems. My heart sank. Each behavior I read added to my apprehension.*

4. Difficulty mixing with other children. *He doesn't just have difficulty mixing. He doesn't mix at all with other children.*

5. Gesturing to show needs. *He doesn't do much of anything to show his needs.* I nervously tapped my pen against the table.

6. No fear of real dangers. *What two-year-old child has fear of danger?*

7. Acting as if deaf. *He does this.*

8. Standoffish manner. *He doesn't pay any attention to the kids in the church nursery. It's as if they don't exist.*

9. Resistance to learning. *He doesn't even like Sesame Street. I'd call that resistance to learning.*

I continued talking to myself, my spirit dropping further into despair.

10. Sustained odd play. I searched my memory. *I wonder if nonexistent appropriate play falls in this category.*

11. Marked physical over activity. *He doesn't have this.*

12. Inappropriate attachment to objects.
*He doesn't have this either.*
13. Inappropriate laughing and giggling.
*Oh, no. I remember a few times in the car, he laughed for no reason.*
14. Spinning of objects. I couldn't remember this happening often. *He did like to spin the beads at the pediatrician's office.*
15. Rocking movements or hand flapping. I gritted my teeth. *He flaps his hands.*

My eyes scanned ahead, and the clamp on my heart tightened. The next one on the list scared me the most.
16. Sparse, meaningless, or echo speech. This one I dreaded most of all. Without speech, how could Jeremy survive in this world? Would this disability forever change my son's world and my family? How was I going to cope with this?

# CHAPTER TWO:
# GRIEF AND GETTING A GRIP

I sat at the dining table, holding my head in my hands. Tears streamed down my face. I heard my husband's car pull into the driveway, so I went to the door to meet him. We held each other as I poured out the story. His grief-stricken face mirrored my own despair.

Had I done something to cause this? Then I remembered the experience in the car on the way to Austin when God had seemed to speak to me His peace and comfort. I wasn't to blame for Jeremy's problems. The thought helped me. The grief was enough to deal with right now without adding guilt on top of that. In God's mercy, he had helped me to work through my possible guilt beforehand. I didn't blame myself.

At work the next day, I told my supervisor. Sympathetically, she offered to send me home. "No, I'm here. I can make it."

Her gaze searched my face and seemed to probe my thoughts. "Sometimes I get the idea some people have everything. It looks like you live the American dream. You're pretty. You have a nice husband and two cute kids. But I guess we all have troubles, no matter who we are. I'm sorry."

At home, fears for the future had become a reality.

My friend Natalie dropped by with her three-year-old son Mark and two-year-old daughter Ashley. As they entered the front door, I looked over at Jeremy. He stood in front of the television with just a diaper on.

Why did Jeremy hate clothes so much? I felt my face heat up.

Jeremy turned and saw our friends. He got on his knees and began banging his head on the floor.

Horrified, I walked over, grabbed his hands, and said close to his face, "No! You will not do that." Then to Natalie I said, "Excuse us for a minute."

Natalie blinked, making an effort to hide her shock and act naturally.

I took Jeremy in the bedroom, dressed him, and went back to make the best of the visit.

As we visited, Mark and Ashley went and played on the small indoor slide we had set up in the spare room.

Jeremy played alone with a toy giraffe, showing no interest in anyone.

After they left, I ached at the contrast between Jeremy and Natalie's children. Her children asked for what they wanted and had defined personalities. The ability to wish and want already existed for her two children. Jeremy couldn't even ask for what he wanted. He couldn't stand to wear clothes. I barely won the struggles to keep a diaper on him at home and clothes when we went out. Maybe I was comparing him too much to others? But I had to have a reference point for his development, right?

The joys of parenthood evaporated, leaving only love and an intense desire to rescue Jeremy from this life of solitude and dependence. Randall was equally determined to help Jeremy. Though he had to work at his business most of the time to provide for our family, he focused with me on Jeremy's needs when he could.

The days that followed didn't get any easier. The information I had read contributed to my discouragement. I also dreaded telling my parents, who had already suffered enough for a lifetime. I arranged to have dinner with them in a restaurant near their home.

I had to tell them. No more procrastinating.

\*\*\*

Later, I sat across from my parents at a restaurant. "Mom. Dad. I need to tell you something,"

They smiled back at me. Though Mother was in her seventies, her brown hair still had less gray than that of many people in their fifties. Dad wore a classy, blue shirt that matched his eyes and reflected his good taste in clothes.

"We thought something was up when Randall and the kids didn't come with you," Mother said.

"You know I've been worried about why Jeremy isn't talking yet, and why he doesn't seem to understand what I say. I took him to an appointment with a child development specialist."

I paused and braced myself inwardly, trying to keep my emotions in check. I needed to be strong for them. "She said she believes Jeremy is autistic." There, I finally said the dreadful words.

"Is the doctor sure, Karen?" my dad asked. "Jeremy seems just fine to me. Doctors can be wrong sometimes."

"Dad, I don't think the doctor is wrong. Jeremy's not interested in interacting with people. He has a way of playing that isn't normal. Jeremy may never talk. Leading a normal life may be impossible. There is a whole list of problems we will have to deal with."

Pausing to see how they took my news, and finding that they were doing well, I said, "It breaks my heart that he may never sing with other children and say 'Mommy, I love you.' What kind of life can he have? I want him to marry some day and have a normal life, not be constantly watched out for. But unless God heals him, he will always have to depend on someone."

I twisted a strand of hair and continued. "He may never be all right. Randall and I will be looking after him the rest of our lives. And when we die, Jennifer will have to look after him. The doctor says there is very little we can do for him. Would you pray that God will heal him?"

I waited to see if Mom or Dad would break down. Instead, they sat serenely. Their deep faith in God radiated from their faces. "Karen, we will pray. God won't leave you now," Mother said. I sighed. This was my mom who had committed to pray an hour a day for nine years in order to see my oldest sister come to salvation. I knew Mother meant it when she said she would pray for Jeremy.

"Thanks for your prayers. Maybe if we pray enough, he'll be healed. It's ridiculous to give up on a child so young."

Mother had helped pray me through troubles in the past. Reassurance settled over me. If anyone needed a prayer warrior during a catastrophe, I'd recommend my mother anytime.

Why had I worried about my parents? Didn't I know how they reacted to hard times by now? Their unwavering faith in God had held me many times. The intense grief and despair in my heart eased slightly because they shared the load.

On the drive home, I cried about the inevitable outcome for my son. Did the future hold any happiness for us?

\*\*\*

I arrived home, parked in the garage, and walked into the kitchen.

Randall came into the kitchen from the hallway. "Jeremy is still awake if you want to go in and say goodnight."

Jeremy was lying on the bed with his eyes open when I walked into his room. He looked like an angel in his blue pajamas that intensified the blue of his eyes. My gaze lovingly traced his adorable face. "Honey, I've come in to pray for you before you go to sleep."

So often in the past, he hadn't understood what I said, so I didn't expect a response. But as I knelt to pray, he got up off the bed and knelt with me. That moment of connection he made into our world was extraordinary for him. It was a ray of hope for me. He stayed there as I prayed, and when I finished, he got up and climbed back into his bed. Tears ran down my face, as I gave my son a hug. "Precious, I'm going to do everything in my power to rescue you from this disability. Nothing will stop me. There has to be hope somewhere. If there is, I will find it." I whispered more to myself than to him.

My promise to Jeremy led our family on a rescue mission to give Jeremy a future, but it would come at a tremendous price.

# CHAPTER THREE:

# LOOKING FOR WHAT IS SUCCESSFUL

A t first we craved information on autism. Then the information turned into a barrage of facts and conflicting views. Whom should we listen to?

I sat next to my husband one evening as we did our bedtime reading. I would read a story about a parent dealing with an autistic child, and then I'd stop and cry.

"I don't know if I can research autism yet, Randall. I'm just too heartbroken." Tears ran down my face.

"What else can we do? We have to find something that will help Jeremy."

"I know," I whispered. I pointed to the story of an autistic child who was mentally retarded in parts of his development and a genius in other areas. "Will Jeremy be like this child when he grows up? This boy's mother kept coming up with reasons why he couldn't talk until he was so old intervention was difficult. I feel like someone threw a million keys in my living room, and I'm supposed to find the ones that open the doors to solve Jeremy's problems."

Randall's forehead furrowed. "I know. I feel the same way."

Then I looked down at the stack of material we had collected. "At least now we're finding good sources of information."

Randall nodded. "And I found out there's a support group for parents with autistic children. We can go to their next meeting."

"Okay, sounds good." I looked down at my reading material. "Here's something interesting. A man named Dr. Rimland and his wife didn't know what was wrong with their son, back in the days when the medical profession said the mother was to blame for her child being autistic. He later wrote a book about autism that changed the medical profession's opinions (Rimland, 1964). I'm sure glad we don't have to work through that sort of stigma. They believe now that autism is caused by a neurological disorder."

While we read and struggled with Jeremy's diagnosis, his condition grew progressively worse. He slid more and more into his own world. He no longer acknowledged Randall or Jennifer. I feared I would lose the connection between him and me. His link with me seemed the only link left that connected him to the rest of the world.

Strangers began to notice that something was wrong. One day in the grocery store, the cashier said to Jeremy, "Hi, young man. What's your name?"

Jeremy only flapped his hands in his peculiar way and said nothing.

The cashier gave him an odd look, clearly uncomfortable with Jeremy's behavior.

"He's not talking yet," I said, attempting to smooth things over. Smiling in spite of the clerk's discomfort, I acted like nothing out of the ordinary had occurred.

Driving home, I wondered if Jeremy could understand what I said. If he did, he might really believe he couldn't talk. I decided I wouldn't say he couldn't talk any more in front of him. Instead, I'd find excuses to tell him he could talk. Whether it helped or not, it couldn't hurt.

Our research continued, as did my prayers that God would heal him. I told my sister one day, desperate for my family and friends to pray for Jeremy's healing. "Pray that God will heal Jeremy."

"Maybe we can pray that God will do a gradual healing. We can pray first for good eye-contact," Mary said.

It didn't sound good enough to me. I yearned to wake up one morning and find Jeremy completely cured. If I received such assurance, I would thank God for healing him and go on, just believing. But so far I had no such assurance from God.

A thought ran through my mind. *Look for what's successful!* Surely God was planting this thought in my mind.

How simple, but profound. This thought was what I needed to hear at that moment. It inspired me to begin a campaign. At every opportunity, I picked other people's brains. Parents. Professionals. Anyone who might know something that would help Jeremy. One of the main questions I asked was, "What were the results of the intervention you tried?" Answers to that question disappointed me on more than one occasion.

I wanted to hear from God, "Your son is healed," but I did not. Looking for what's successful was the closest I could come to any answer from God, so I plowed through data, cried, asked questions, and continued to pray.

When Jeremy was two years and eight months old, I took him to the local Early Childhood Intervention group that the child development specialist referred me to. They were kind and promised to test him and then commit to some therapy time based on his need.

I waited for them to tell me how many hours they could give Jeremy.

"We are going to give you two speech sessions a week and one of occupational therapy session." I frowned. Instinctively I knew this would never be enough. I had hoped for some sort of daily therapy.

Then I browsed the sheet that described their profile of Jeremy. My gaze landed on the line for expressive language. It said eight months old. My heart lunged. I mentally calculated Jeremy's age. This couldn't be right.

His overall communication developmental age was one year old. The ache in my heart increased.

I read the rest. His daily living skills ranged from five months old to fifteen months old. Socialization was at ten months.

*This can't be.* I wanted to reject the news. It was worse than I feared.

He was about two years behind developmentally.

I felt the gap in his development was as distant as the time it took for light to travel from a remote star to the earth—impossible.

In the days that followed, I appealed to everyone I knew to pray for Jeremy. I was so desperate I asked people who didn't even believe in prayer to pray because my sense of urgency was so intense.

I remember calling Sue, a friend in another state. I poured out my needs and asked for prayer. I knew she believed in prayer. I could feel her hesitate and then she said, "I know I have never been through anything like this, but I want you to know I'm sorry."

"Thank you. Someone that I read recently wrote that they believed there are only two things more serious than autism—cerebral palsy and Down's syndrome. I'm not sure this is true, but it's an indicator of how serious autism is. This situation with Jeremy being autistic is one thing I thought would never happen to me. I thought when you followed God's will the best you know how, nothing like this would happen."

"I know what you mean."

"As far as I know, Randall and I have done nothing wrong, so this situation must be like the blind man in the Bible. You remember that story? The one where the disciples asked Jesus, 'Why was this man born blind? Was it because of his sins or his parents' sins?' And Jesus said, 'It was neither, it was for the glory of God.' I have to believe God will work this out for the good. I must not accept blame where there is none. It doesn't really matter how or why Jeremy has this disorder. It's here, and all I want to know is how to fix it."

I didn't want to accept and cope with this problem—I wanted a cure for it. Whether God provided it through miraculous healing or through other people, I wanted an answer to my prayer. When I heard stories of families who resigned themselves to the fact that there was nothing they could do about autism and instead put their efforts into coping skills. I couldn't make that decision for Jeremy—certainly not until we tried any reasonable intervention.

At the first autism support group Randall and I attended, I soaked up all the information I could. All the mothers seemed stressed to the breaking point, and each couple worked as hard as anyone I had ever known to help their children. Many times, Randall and I came away from support meetings with helpful information. When Randall found something useful, he passed on the material to me. Even before we had entered into this crisis with Jeremy, I had quit my full-time job to be with him more. I had no idea it would be such a wise decision. Both Randall and I put our whole-hearted effort into helping Jeremy. Realistically, Randall had to spend the majority of his time with his work, making the money to support the family and the cost of therapy.

We continued to attend support group meetings. I noticed members of the group were thrilled by every little glimpse of development in their child. To me helping our children learn seemed like riding a stationary exercise bike—after peddling three miles we found ourselves in the same spot.

"I heard Dr. Kotsanis speak recently. He has helped lots of autistic people. We are going to have George tested for allergies," Linda, one of the parents attending that night, said.

That sounded good because during my reading I discovered many autistic children have severe food allergies.

"My son knows his colors and letters. His diagnosis is PDD (Pervasive Developmental Disorder)," said another mother. She said this as if PDD was less severe than autism. I questioned whether PDD was an improvement over autism. When I read about or met children with a PDD diagnosis, it looked the same as autism to me. Though having a PDD diagnosis sounded like a milder disability than autism—was it? Her child had a severe verbal and social impairment. I thought of our situation—what if my son had fewer autistic behaviors from the list but ended up with each behavior being more severe? It would gain nothing to have a PDD diagnosis versus autism. In our case, Jeremy's speech was severely lacking, so even if he had no other indicators of autism than having a language deficit, we would still have trouble. And he did have other symptoms.

Later, sadly, my instincts about the child with PDD proved correct. His problems grew worse. His parents spent many hours trying to console him, and at night it was difficult for him to sleep. He lost all knowledge of colors and letters his mother had been so proud of, and he had almost no verbal skills. It was heartbreaking.

I learned from that family's experience. I realized I must not worry about how to label Jeremy's disability. Dealing with what was wrong was most important. No matter what the rare encouraging action Jeremy had, he was still autistic and faced a grim unknown future. That would keep me researching and working.

Our support group talked as if they hoped to find the miracle cure, but it seemed clear to me we had found only small solutions up to that point. Could we hope to find answers that provided more than subtle, almost indiscernible, improvements in our children? I longed for answers that improved quality of life for Jeremy and the other children. What my heart cried out for most of all was—a cure. Yet I listened intently at the meetings because if the interventions they discussed were reasonable, I wanted to try them.

Most of the parents talked about using behavior modification when dealing with their children, so I came home to read more about it. I knew spanking didn't work with Jeremy, so I thought behavior modification was worth a try. I had an opportunity to practice my newfound knowledge at bedtime one evening.

"Jeremy, it's time to go to bed," I said.

My request caused immediate crying and resistance.

I walked over and took his hand. He dragged his weight in the opposite direction as I attempted to walk him to the bedroom. I acted as if the tantrum didn't affect me in any way or even exist. "No, come."

Since he didn't obey, I picked him up and placed him on the floor in the right direction. "Yes, that way."

He resisted once more, and I repeated my action. Amazingly, he caught on and walked on his own to the bedroom. As he walked, I praised him to reinforce good behavior.

It worked.

Later I returned to the living room.

"You did that well," Randall said.

I smiled. "I read that in a book." But learning how to use this technique wasn't as easy as it sounded. Jeremy had a mind of his own. It took months of work and reading to get good enough to use it effectively. Eventually I used this technique to handle Jeremy and to direct his learning.

\*\*\*

We made an appointment with a specialist we had heard about through Linda in our support group. We drove the four-hour trip to Grapevine, Texas.

When the nurse called Jeremy's name, Randall, Jeremy, and I walked into the examination room. After a short wait, a distinguished-looking, olive-skinned man entered the room.

He introduced himself as Dr. Kotsanis and began asking questions about Jeremy.

We told Dr. Kotsanis our concerns. "My wife and I would like to have Jeremy tested for food allergies," Randall said.

"Yes, we can do that here." Then Dr. Kotsanis proceeded to tell us about all the treatments he gave his autistic patients. Though he exuded sincerity and enthusiasm, I saw no evidence of a cure here.

We listened to him in a selective way—picking and choosing what we thought would help Jeremy.

As we left, we agreed to have Jeremy tested for yeast levels, irritable bowel syndrome, parasitic activity, and food allergies. On the drive home, we discussed the visit.

"You know, I never thought of myself as an alternative medicine kind of person before this, but when traditional medicine has offered no help, what else can we do?" I said. I looked over at Randall as he steered the car onto the highway. He pressed his lips into a line.

"Why is everything a thousand dollars?" Randall asked.

"I know what you mean. I don't know how much to trust him. I don't think he's just after the money. He really believes in what he's doing. The tests Dr. Kotsanis will run may not be a cure, but if these treatments help Jeremy physically—they are worth it. Jeremy needs to be as healthy as possible so he can learn."

We rode in silence a few miles. Randall said, "When you read some of these testimonies about kids who have undergone some of these treatments, they act so excited, like it's a cure-all. It's a little misleading because the bottom line is—they are still autistic."

"I understand, but at least the treatments improve some aspects of their lives," I said.

"Oh, I agree. It's worth it if nothing else to improve quality of life."

***

Janelle, the speech therapist from the early childhood intervention group, arrived the next week to start her routine visits with Jeremy.

"Jeremy, look," Janelle said. She made sounds into a colorful toy microphone that amplified her voice. Jeremy took the microphone from her and proceeded to bang the toy on the floor.

Grabbing the microphone back from Jeremy, she rescued the toy by placing it into a large canvas bag. She then brought out a dollhouse and matching dolls and handed him the boy doll.

Jeremy took the boy doll and put him in the dollhouse.

Focusing attention back to me, Janelle said, "We need to play games with Jeremy that will encourage him to talk. Play therapy might be the answer for Jeremy. Also, I brought you some information about a therapy called Hanen." She handed me the papers, and I scanned the sheet.

"Thank you. I'll look into it." I laid the paper on the table next to me and reached for the other doll. Placing the doll on the toy merry-go-round, I looked at Jeremy and wondered if teaching him play skills would help him talk. So far, giving Jeremy attention had helped, but he still wasn't talking. There must be more that could be done. For a normal child, play activities would stimulate speech, but something was short-circuited with Jeremy's development. I didn't believe any amount of playing would bring the miracle we needed. I longed for a method that would teach Jeremy to talk.

"I'm going to buy a couple of books Randall and I have heard about from our autism support group. One is *Let Me Hear Your Voice* by Catherine Maurice and the other one is *The Sound of a Miracle* by Annabel Stehli," I said to Janelle.

"Let me know what you find out."

I began a reading spree that left me more hopeful than I had been since the day the doctor used the word *autism* when discussing Jeremy.

Anxious for feedback from the autism support group, I brought my questions to the next meeting and asked about *The Sound of a Miracle*. "Linda, do you know anything about Auditory Integration Training? I read a book called *The Sound of a Miracle*, and a child was cured from autism through this therapy."

"Yes, we took George to Dr. Kotsanis, who has a trained person in his office to implement the therapy."

"Did it help?"

"Yes, he seems to be a little better."

My heart sunk in disappointment. This didn't seem to be the answer either. I wanted something dramatic. I wanted to hear *yes, my son talks so much more now* or something equally remarkable. I asked others and heard the same lukewarm responses.

Mentioning Auditory Integration Training therapy to a friend who worked in a health services clinic, I asked, "Have you

33

heard of Auditory Integration Training? It's the therapy used in a book called *The Sound of a Miracle.*"

"I've heard of this, Karen. I understand the mother is disappointed it hasn't helped other children as dramatically as it has her daughter."

"I can imagine. But at least it seems to help some kids. If it improves quality of life, I think it's a good thing."

At another support group meeting one mother said, "We are doing play therapy. A doctor in Maryland is really good at this."

"What's his name?" I asked.

"Dr. Greenspan. I'll give the address and phone number after the meeting."

Hearing of play therapy from two sources, I decided to read the Hanen material I had received from Jeremy's speech therapist. Then I put a call into Dr. Greenspan in Maryland.

# CHAPTER FOUR:

# INFORMATION OVERLOAD

One day, when Janelle came to our home for Jeremy's weekly speech therapy session, we spent time discussing ways to help him.

"Janelle, I've learned about a therapy called Behavioral Intervention started by Dr. Lovaas of UCLA. Lovaas and his colleagues did a scientific study in the 1980s, and found that 47% of the children who go through this therapy, if started around three years old, can become indistinguishable from other children their age (Lovaas, 1987). It's normally a therapy program that takes from two to six years to complete and runs when the child is young. The therapy looks very promising." I said the last part hoping she would pay attention and encourage me on using the therapy for Jeremy.

A frown creased her brow. "I've heard about this therapy. It's harmful, Karen. I don't think you should pursue it."

I frowned back. I didn't understand. What was wrong? "The techniques they are using now have few negative aspects," I said, defending the method. "It's the kind of behavior management that Helen Keller received. It doesn't have to be misused. I don't have to do anything harsh if I don't want to. It isn't as if the children are given shock treatment." I didn't know at the time that all adverse methods had been removed from the Lovaas' therapy approach (called Behavioral Intervention or ABA, Applied Behavioral Analysis). I was beginning to figure out that many professionals were from an old school that cautioned about the old days of shock treatment experiments. Today there was a whole new world of methodology. Now positive reinforcement was used to encourage the child while learning.

The look in her eyes reflected her disbelief in the proposed system.

"I have an extra copy of the book I've been reading. I'll give it to you to read."

With a smile and a "thank you," Janelle left with the book and promised to read it. It was important to me that she gave her approval of the therapy. Somehow not having a professional's encouragement to pursue the therapy was disconcerting. After the door shut, Jennifer took my hand. "Mommy, can I have a friend over?"

"Not today, honey." I gave her a hug and inwardly worried for what seemed like the thousandth time, *is Jennifer receiving the attention she needs?*

How could a six-year-old possibly understand? Could I tell her that all this attention Jeremy received was for her benefit, too? If we didn't help him now—if we didn't conquer this disability now—who would take care of him after Randall and I died? Would Jennifer spend her life caring for her brother? And what would happen when she was gone? Who would care for him then?

I pushed aside my worries about Jennifer and focused on my next task. The time had come to make some phone calls—calls that would give me information on Behavioral Intervention therapy available to parents in Texas. I found the phone number of the New Jersey clinic, a clinic that Dr. Lovaas had started. I called, but they did not have an opening for a year. The news hit me like a blast of cold air.

"I'll be dead by then," I said to the person on the other end of the phone, joking to keep myself from crying. "Where can I find someone to help me? The UCLA clinic just has a recording that says they are not taking out-of-state patients."

"There is another clinic that has been opened in Wisconsin. Would you like that phone number?"

I quickly agreed, and the receptionist gave me the number and hung up. Hope welled in me once again. I dialed the Wisconsin number. The person at the other end of the line gave me information and assured me they could get me on the list but that a workshop could not be scheduled until January. She assured me that I would be contacted at a later date to come up with the exact dates.

That was months down the road! I did some quick mental calculations of Jeremy's age. In January, Jeremy would be three and a half years old. Was starting therapy at that age be soon enough? I knew starting at a young age was critical.

I wished he was starting at three years old. Could six months make that much difference? I had a copy of the study, and I could look up the age of the kids that participated.

Hearing a noise at the back door, I turned to find Randall coming inside. He stopped and waited for me to get off the line. I smiled and finished discussing testing requirements and other steps needed before our first workshop and then hung up.

"I'm so excited. This clinic can take us." A thought entered my mind that caused my excitement to dip. "It still seems so far away. I hope we are starting soon enough to be effective for Jeremy."

"Can we do the therapy on our own?" Randall said. "What books are available?"

"There's not enough information out in books yet. *The Me Book* (Lovaas, 1981) has some of the beginning drills, but it's out of date. I don't think they're doing the therapy that way anymore." (I have since learned that parents can use the book, *Teaching Individuals with Developmental Delays*, by O. Ivar Lovaas for up-to-date information. *The Me Book* is incomplete and out-of-date.)

"What's *The Me Book*?"

"Dr. Lovaas wrote it. I'll see what I can get out of it and start some drills." We walked into the living room as we talked.

Jeremy stood in front of the TV in his diaper. He was getting too old to wear just a diaper.

What was Jeremy getting out of this TV program? He certainly wasn't getting any language from watching. It seemed to contribute more to his disability. I scowled at Jeremy's back and turned to watch my husband leave the room. Did Randall realize Jeremy needed professional help and that I couldn't give it to him? If I hadn't quit my full-time job to spend my time with Jeremy, I don't think I would have noticed the urgent need. I believed Randall would see the whole picture soon. In spite of the fact I was unsure of Randall understanding, our unity and sole aim had been to get intervention for Jeremy. I took this for granted, and I was never disappointed in Randall's support before this. I focused on Jeremy, and Randall focused on supporting the family. Though many times Randall would research and pass the information on to me, the hours of work for Jeremy needed to come from me.

I walked over and turned off the television. Taking Jeremy's hand, I said, "No more TV for now, honey." I led him to his basket of toy cars, picked up one, and said, "Zoom. Look at the car go," then handed him one. He responded, and I was glad. *But what about learning language? This isn't helping enough.* I knew from some of my reading some kids didn't respond at all to playing. Jeremy did, but I asked myself again, was it enough?

I couldn't understand what Jeremy thought about all day long. When we didn't seek him out, he would spend hours staring at the TV or moving toys around. One of his favorite pastimes was marking on the wall. No matter how many times I said no, he still marked on the walls in every room of the house. He also liked to pull books out of bookshelves. I knew it went way beyond the normal toddler misbehaving. It was connected to his disability.

My husband walked in the room. "Karen, did you happen to ask the Wisconsin clinic if there is anyone doing therapy in Texas? Maybe you could visit them."

"No, I didn't."

"Give me the number, and I'll ask them."

Randall reached for the number and left to make the phone call.

It was time to start supper, but I wanted to work with Jeremy. He just stagnated when I didn't work with him. But how could I spend every moment of every day with him? My heart ached, and the hopelessness of the situation overwhelmed me once again.

The days followed with a pattern of spending as much time as possible with Jeremy and studying the small amount of information we had on ABA. I wanted to try the therapy on Jeremy. Though I hoped to get a call soon to set up our first workshop for Jeremy, I didn't want to waste any time.

Janelle wanted me to send Jeremy to the public preschool program. Only kids who were behind developmentally were allowed. Maybe the preschool program would help me implement the therapy. I learned he needed about forty hours a week of one-on-one, and we needed to start soon. He was three, and I was anxious not to lose the opportunity to help him now. Randall and I had a tendency to procrastinate. I knew this from experience that several months could pass, and we wouldn't accomplish anything. The study made it plain that starting therapy at a young age was one of the decisive factors in the therapy.

Randall's call to the Wisconsin clinic resulted in finding a family in a nearby city using the therapy. In the meantime, I visited the public school preschool class Jeremy would attend. Driving over, I worried this might be the wrong decision. *What if they are unwilling to help me? What if Jeremy gets into special education and never gets out?*

I walked into the classroom with trepidation. The teacher had all the right qualities. She was loving, professional, attentive, and more. But something wasn't right for me. The kids in her class were not severely handicapped, but I got the impression they would never go to a normal classroom. Did any kids graduate to a regular classroom? From my research, it looked as if an autistic child rarely if ever caught up developmentally as a result of special education class. I remember the words in the autism literature—lifelong, incurable, and incapacitating. My brain would forever hold those grim words in memory, and my heart cried out because of the hopelessness of it all. Special education had been around a long time. I didn't want a lifetime of special education for him. But was this something I had to accept? Was it true that once he was behind other children his age he would always be behind? I didn't like the idea of having such low expectations for Jeremy.

I knew parents of autistic children who had accepted and coped wonderfully, and I knew God could provide the grace and strength to handle this. But I rebelled at the thought. My child was three years old—must I accept the status quo and give up? The likelihood of Jeremy recovering through the public school special education system was small. No matter how much I appreciated and respected the dedicated teachers and aides of the public school, this was the blunt truth—at least in the case of autism.

I asked the teacher and the aides if they had ever seen or heard of an autistic child who recovered in the public school system. The answer was no.

Did traditional special education and speech therapy produce any recovered autistic individuals? Was there even a rare individual who existed who had come from as far behind as Jeremy was and made it to normal functioning? I began to cry right there in the classroom. The adults in the classroom seemed embarrassed for me, but I couldn't help it. And I didn't care. Jeremy was my baby. He was three years old, and I felt as if I was putting him into the black hole of the special education system. I thought he might never come out. Surely there was another way. If we started down this road, would we drop our plans for implementing ABA therapy? If special education was what he needed and all he could accomplish, fine, but I wanted to give him the chance to do more. I used to regard special ed children as having a learning disability that could never be overcome. I had believed there was no way to ever compensate for their deficits.

But I wanted more for my own son. What a difference being a parent makes.

After the visit to the classroom, the special education group met with me to discuss plans for Jeremy.

\*\*\*

That evening I sat with my husband after dinner. "How did the special ed visit go, Karen?"

"Depressing. I don't really want to put Jeremy in a special ed class. I'm afraid he will never come out."

"Was the teacher nice? How did the meeting go regarding his individual education plan?"

"The teacher was really nice, but I don't think Jeremy will get enough one-on-one attention. At the meeting, several people from the special ed department came to work up a plan for him. I told them about the ABA therapy and how successful it sounded, but my impression is they're going to do exactly what they've always done. They smiled and said, 'That's nice,' but they didn't schedule anything I suggested. I don't see how other parents get what they want for their kids."

"How much ST (speech therapy) and OT (occupational therapy) is he going to get?"

"Only one ST a week and one OT a month."

Randall grimaced. His lips formed a thin line. "That's not going to make enough difference."

I nodded. "I agree. I don't understand how this small amount of work is going to make the impact it needs in his life. If the local football team practiced once a week, could they win any football games? It's ridiculous how little time they think is needed to teach an autistic child to talk. For these kids it's like learning a second language or worse. It doesn't come naturally."

# CHAPTER FIVE:
## THIS IS LIFE NOW, KAREN

One Sunday at church, I paused in the large meeting room where our congregation worshiped every Sunday and talked with one of my best friends, Kelly. Trying to keep an eye on Jeremy, I kept turning my head as I talked. The side door of the room led out into a street. Afraid he would escape and get hurt, I watched him every minute.

"I really think I've found the therapy that will mean something for Jeremy," I said. "For some reason this therapy has stirred up lots of controversy. But it's the most successful I've found of the therapy approaches I've researched. Forty-seven percent of the kids, if started young enough, become indistinguishable from their peers. Dr. Lovaas of UCLA has worked on a teaching approach since the sixties. It helps teach speech, social, and academic skills for autistic children."

"What does 'indistinguishable from their peers' mean?" Kelly asked.

"It just means that you can't tell them apart from normal developing children after the therapy period is over."

"Have you started working with Jeremy?"

"I have done a little work with him, but I don't know what I'm doing. I'm concerned during the teaching sessions that I work him too long and too hard. I hope I can hire a consultant."

All of a sudden I couldn't see Jeremy and began to panic. I ran to the door and looked around.

"Mommy." I heard my daughter call out. I turned to find Jennifer leading Jeremy by the hand.

"Mommy, Jeremy was running out into the street so I got him."

"Oh, honey. Thank you, precious." My fears were justified. I had to guard Jeremy every split-second of the day. Kneeling down I drew both my children into an embrace. Love swelled in my heart as little boy sweat rubbed against one side of my face and Jennifer's silky hair tickled the other side. Was this the beginning of a lifetime of watching out for Jeremy? Not just at age three, but age ten, fifteen, thirty?

From that moment on, I knew I would have to be more alert to Jeremy's every movement. Other three-year-olds had to be watched carefully but not quite so intensely. He had no fear of danger. Jeremy was developmentally about one year old, but his gross motor skills were the same as those of any other three-year-old child.

Though Jeremy was too heavy for me, I tried holding him while I continued talking with Kelly.

"I want to finish our conversation. Where were we?"

Kelly turned to me with a sad expression on her face. "You know, I have a friend, Marta, with an autistic son. Her son's name is Joseph, and he sets the table for the meals. Would you be interested in getting together with Marta?"

"No, not at this point, thank you though. I need to find someone making big breakthroughs," I said with a sigh.

My instincts told me that talking with Marta would lead nowhere. From my support group I already knew of too many parents who found unrealistic hope in the small achievements of their children. Sadly, I found out a few months later that Marta and her husband had to have Joseph institutionalized.

I wanted to help my son in a dramatic way—I wanted him to talk and not just cope. I wanted a cure for his disability. Hopefully, ABA therapy would work for Jeremy. Once again I was motivated to get started.

Setting Jeremy down, I started to tell Kelly what our hopes were for Jeremy when my husband walked up and told us the potluck dinner was being served. I managed to keep Jeremy with me as I went through the line and dished out plates of food for both of us. When we sat down, I dove into the food, hoping to finish my meal before Jeremy took off for destinations unknown.

I ached to talk, visit with others and relax, but soon found myself following Jeremy around the large meeting room while trying to balance my plate of food and eat at the same time. I had lost count of the number of times I hadn't been able to sit down and eat Sunday dinner. Trying to make the best of it, I continued trailing Jeremy past rows of now empty chairs toward the platform.

Robert, my brother-in-law, walked by us and gave me a friendly hello. He continued toward the serving table where he got in line with my sister, Mary. I heard him in the distance telling Mary, "Karen doesn't have a life. She—" His voice faded as I followed Jeremy to the opposite end of the room.

I guess I didn't have a life. It must be bad if even Robert had noticed. Normally I would be feeling sorry for myself, but between the food and the sympathy expressed by Robert, my heart felt a little lighter. *Face it, Karen. This is your life now.*

I looked down at Jeremy. He was crossing his eyes. It was something I had noticed before. But this wasn't a case of a mischievous ten-year-old boy trying to irritate his sister. This behavior belonged to a three-year-old boy who was oblivious to the people around him and was slipping into a world of his own. This was atypical, and I didn't like it. The last time I had seen him cross his eyes I had made up a plan on how to handle him, if he should do it again.

Leaning down, I got right in his face, pointed my finger at him and sternly said, "No eye-crossing." The direction needed to be clear and concise so that he would understand.

He must have understood, because immediately he stopped crossing his eyes. In the next few minutes I had to tell him two more times and each time he stopped.

I hoped this helped. If this worked and I was doing the right thing, this behavior should fade and never come back.

A few minutes later Randall was ready to go, so we all loaded in the car.

"Today..." Randall started a sentence and abruptly stopped. The frown on his face got my attention.

"What?"

Randall started again. "Today I happened to be in the men's room when Doug was with his three-year-old son. They were having a very sophisticated conversation. Jeremy isn't even close to basic one-year-old words, much less a conversation."

"I know what you mean. No only is he not conversing, but he seems to be losing ground. We are throwing intervention at him, but we don't know what we're doing. It's not enough."

"I know."

Sadness covered me like a blanket.

\*\*\*

The next day Dr. Greenspan from Maryland returned my phone call. Dr. Greenspan advocated play therapy so we had a lengthy discussion, and I was impressed with the genuine concern he conveyed to me during our conversation. At the end of the call, I decided to ask my most important question.

"What kind of success have you had with play therapy, Dr. Greenspan?"

"Play therapy can help significantly."

I didn't want a vague answer.

Trying to pin him down, I asked, "How many autistic kids have you seen recover?" I didn't care at the moment how scientific the answer. Was it one, ten, fifteen, or none?

Again he answered in vague, general terms. My heart sank. *This isn't for Jeremy.*

I had spent hours playing with Jeremy, but it was like going one step forward and two steps back. Playing wasn't teaching him to talk or form sentences.

Hanging up the phone, I leaned against the kitchen counter. "Lord," I prayed aloud. "I don't know if I can do this. If ABA therapy is the answer for Jeremy, we have to give him forty hours a week of one-on-one concentrated effort. I thought when my youngest became three years old I'd have some relief. I don't know if I can continue to give that much."

*I did.* A still small voice seemed to say.

Was this God speaking to me? This seemed outside of my own thought processes.

Yes, I thought to myself, Jesus gave His whole life—not just at the end when He gave His life on the cross, but the times He taught, healed, and talked to the people even when he was tired. He mentored his disciples. He came to give. If the Lord poured out His all for me, why couldn't I give the next few years to my son?

This gave me hope. I could do this with God's help.

# CHAPTER SIX:

# THE GOOD, THE BAD, AND THE

# BEAUTIFUL

---

"Ee... eek!" Screaming came from the hall. From my seat in the large Sunday school room, I couldn't see the source of the screaming.

Randall had made some phone calls and found an ABA workshop for us to attend in Austin, Texas. The workshop was all for one four-year-old girl, Kayla. Her parents, Melissa and Ron, were holding the Saturday session of Kayla's workshop in a large church room to accommodate the people interested in watching.

The screaming grew closer, until in ran a wild-eyed girl who needed no introduction. Though a physically beautiful child, Kayla clearly had something wrong with her.

Randall sat next to me, along with another set of parents, several women who were training to be therapists, and a few professionals: speech therapists, occupational therapists, and a psychologist.

Kayla ran by my chair. Like a wild animal, she steered clear of people in the room, never giving eye contact to anyone. *Would Jeremy eventually be like this?* Kayla was approaching her fifth birthday. I now understood Melissa's urgency in setting up a learning program for her. Avoiding her parents' attempts to make her cooperate, Kayla turned, allowing me the full view of her face. Her beauty astonished me. *Whoa.* Her eyes were like Jeremy's—eyes so incredible it was like heaven looking out. I had noticed this look in a few other autistic children as well.

After a few more minutes, Ron picked her up and gently placed her on one of the chairs at a small table where a bucket and some blocks had been placed. The young consultant, Crystal, who looked to be right out of college, tried to control Kayla and teach the group at the same time.

Crystal positioned herself and Kayla where they could both have a good view of the table. Picking up a block, Crystal placed it in the bucket and said, "Do this."

Kayla started screaming again. Crystal said again, "Do this," then took Kayla's hand, used it to pick up a block, and put it in the bucket. "Good."

Crystal made four more simple requests and rewarded Kayla with verbal praise for every correct response. Then she told Kayla, "Go play."

Turning to us, Crystal explained, "You have to start out simple. This has to be rewarding to the child. We give a request in a short, simple manner. Then reward her for each correct response. Eventually, Kayla will get the idea that it's more fun and rewarding to learn and respond."

Crystal expounded on some technical terms used in the therapy and on some ways to handle the drills and behavior problems. Glancing at Melissa and the women training to be therapists, she said, "You need to find what is most rewarding for Kayla, whether it's verbal praise, food, or whatever. When she gives the right response, you reward her. If she gives the wrong answer, just give an informational 'no,' nothing negative."

Crystal had barely begun her explanation when the woman next to me interrupted. "I don't see what good this will do. I believe this is harmful to Kayla." The woman scowled, her chin tilted up, her nose up in the air. She continued to dominate the floor—fifteen, then twenty minutes.

I wished Melissa, Ron, or the consultant would tell her to be quiet. This workshop was costing hundreds, maybe thousands, of dollars for Melissa and Ron. Her attitude seemed to say, *How dare you question me? I'm a professional. This therapy approach is beneath me.* She came across like someone criticizing an architect for a plan while only looking at a window and not the whole building.

I wanted to get up and tell her that she hadn't even heard the complete introduction to the therapy approach yet, much less listened to what it was all about.

Why was she so against this type of therapy? What could hurt a child to learn to answer some questions at a table? With the exception of Crystal, why did every professional in the room seem to be on Ms. Know-It-All's side? Why wouldn't the woman wait to see what it was all about?

I longed to tell her my conviction that the method Crystal was demonstrating was helping children and that, with consistent work, Kayla would stop having tantrums and start learning just as Helen Keller had. I had much to learn myself, but I did know enough to want to hear Crystal's whole presentation before I passed judgment.

Finally I couldn't stand it. Attempting to be as diplomatic as possible, I said, "I'm a parent of an autistic child. And I want my child to learn and change. I want to break through to him."

Melissa said, "Me, too. That's why I'm having this workshop." Then everyone began to talk at once, and the session turned into utter chaos. I saw the consultant say something to Ron. Then he stepped forward and dismissed the group for lunch.

After Randall and I left for the restaurant, I said, "I feel so sorry for Melissa and Ron. That woman is wasting their time. Do you realize how much this workshop is costing them? They are paying for the consultant's time, travel expenses, and all the people hired to work with her."

"Crystal should have told her to be quiet."

"How can she? It wouldn't be polite to say anything since Melissa and Ron were the ones who invited her to the workshop. They should be the ones to ask the woman to be quiet."

"When we have our workshop for Jeremy, we are not having any professionals," Randall said.

"I know one or two that are open-minded about the therapy. I'd really like them to know about it. Can I invite professionals if they are sympathetic toward our therapy approach?"

Randall turned into the restaurant parking lot, parked the car then turned to me. "Okay, but we need to be cautious about whom to invite to our workshops."

We went into the restaurant, and after getting our food we sat down to eat. Picking up a French fry, I pointed it at Randall as if to emphasize a point. "Did you hear the conversation I was having with that mom visiting the workshop? She and her husband have an autistic son about three years old. They are thinking about starting therapy for him soon."

"Yeah. And did you hear the dad say he didn't want to do it because he didn't want people coming in and out of their house all the time?" The tone of Randall's voice conveyed his disbelief.

"Really! Is that why he left early?" I replied, equally amazed. "It seems like such a small sacrifice to make for your child. Doing without a little privacy now and then seems like nothing. I've heard people say they can't come up with the money, which is understandable, but this? Amazing."

"Yeah, I know. Did you hear that Dan in the autism support group is putting off doing therapy for his little girl because he wants to go back to school? His older kids are in junior high and high school, and he's been waiting to do this for a few years."

"We shouldn't be too hard on him. It is a big sacrifice of time and resources to do this. Maybe he doesn't realize what it will mean for their future to put effort into his child early when it can have the most impact on her."

"Speaking of resources, did you do the cost calculations on how much this therapy program will cost?"

"Uh-huh," I mumbled, trying to think of a way to avoid this conversation. *Oh, well, here goes.* "It looks like it will be at least $20,000 to $30,000 for one year, and we need—"

"What!" Randall interrupted my explanation. "Can't we figure out a way to do the therapy ourselves so we don't have to spend so much money?"

I could feel an argument coming. I fought to keep my voice at an even tone, to keep it from going into a high-pitched whine. "As I was saying, we need to keep this up for about two to six years. I've heard some say it cost about $70,000 a year. I know it looks like we can't do this financially. But maybe we can borrow money. I'm including everything in my estimate—consultant fees for workshops, salaries for the therapists we hire, etc. And no, I can't do this by myself. I've tried, and there just isn't a complete guide for everything I need to know. I don't know how to teach conversation or any of the harder drills. We need a workshop specifically designed for Jeremy."

Randall opened his mouth to say something, but I glanced at my watch and said, "Time to get back. We're going to be late. The session is going to start in five minutes."

\*\*\*

A couple of days later, I called Melissa. "I appreciate so much you and your husband allowing us to come to Kayla's workshop. How are y'all doing? Are you doing any of the therapy yourself?"

"We're doing okay," Melissa said. "I have people coming in and out, off and on all day, but I'm not doing any of the therapy myself. I have plenty to do without scheduling myself."

"What did you think of Crystal? Is she good?"

"She's okay. She seems too young though."

*What's that got to do with anything?* I thought to myself, but I said, "Crystal has done her internship with Dr. Lovaas of UCLA and has a degree in Psychology at the University of Wisconsin-Madison. And most importantly she has hours of experience in a successful therapy approach. I think she knows her stuff." *I guess time will tell.*

"Yeah, maybe. Hey, I'm sorry. I have to get off the phone. I'll catch you later."

# CHAPTER SEVEN:

# PUBLIC SCHOOL AND TEACCH

Worry and anxiety over Jeremy's future dominated my thoughts, keeping me awake at night. One particular night, I gave up trying to sleep. I glanced at the clock. *Ugh, 2 a.m.* Quietly, so as not to wake Randall, I got up and picked up a blanket and headed for the living room.

On the way, I peeked into the kids' rooms to check on them. Everything looked fine in Jennifer's room so I went on to Jeremy's. I didn't see him anywhere. Almost every night he ended up sleeping somewhere other than his bed so I wasn't alarmed. Sometimes he slept on the floor next to his bed, sometimes under his bed, sometimes on the living room floor. It disturbed me when he didn't sleep in his bed. Was this inconsistency a sign of a mind not at rest? Did other parents experience this behavior from their children? It just didn't seem healthy.

Walking further into his room, I looked under the bed and around the floor but didn't see him. I checked the living room, still no Jeremy.

Dread filled my heart. I had heard stories of autistic children who would run out of the house and wander the neighborhood. Had he somehow gotten out of the house? I ran back to Jeremy's room. This time I turned on the light. Maybe he was under the bed, and I just hadn't seen him.

Getting on my hands and knees, I looked under his bed again, then I reached out my hand and felt. Finally. My hand hit something over near the wall. Relief swept over me. He had positioned himself in the far corner against the wall. I struggled to grab his leg, and then I pulled him out.

Putting him back on the bed, I stared down at my still sleeping son. I wanted so much for him to be happy, to talk, play, and sing with other children. I lightly placed my hand on his foot. Why did love have to hurt so much? A renewed determination filled me.

*Lord*, I prayed, walking to the living room, *please, help us. We've got to do something. Surely you hear the prayers of a mother in a special way. When you were on earth, Jesus, you had compassion on the widow who lost her son. You raised him from the dead and gave him back to his mother. Please send me reassurance, Lord.* I begged and pleaded and cried. I knew God heard me and saw my tears, but I didn't know how he would answer.

Sensing something, I looked up from praying. Randall stood right inside the door. "What's wrong, Karen?"

Getting up I walked into his arms, and he held me. "I'm so worried about Jeremy. What is to become of him and us? How bad is this going to get? I want to pray until I get an answer."

Putting his cheek against mine, he continued to hold me. After a few moments of silent mutual grief, he whispered, "We both need some sleep, hon'. Let's go back to bed."

Randall's concern for Jeremy showed up even at night— he unconsciously ground his teeth together in his sleep. The dentist had given him teeth guards to wear to protect his teeth. Lying down, I listened for him to begin the even breathing of sleep. Exhaustion caught up with me, and I too faded into a deep sleep.

***

Fortunately, Randall and I were equally committed to helping Jeremy, but I worried that Randall would start depending on the public school or speech therapy to rescue Jeremy from his developmental delays.

Jeremy had started the pre-school special ed program at the public school with a nice teacher, but it didn't matter how wonderful Jeremy's teacher was—it just wasn't enough. The attention he received was like using a bucket of water on a forest fire. At the rate Jeremy was progressing in the class, he would never catch up with others his age. I guessed they didn't think he was capable of catching up, or they had to spread their resources over too many students.

While I was visiting Jeremy's class one day, the teacher pointed out that Jeremy was interacting with another boy in the class. The boy would scramble through a child-size maze, and Jeremy would laugh at the boy's silliness as he scurried through one of the conduits. No conversation would accompany the interchange between the boys.

Momentarily, the cute interchange lifted my heart. But then I reminded myself that though his behavior might be meaningful and great, I'd learned from watching and listening to other parents of autistic children that parents tend to get false hope from isolated appropriate behaviors. One instance of interacting didn't make up for all the other things lacking in his development. Most importantly, Jeremy needed to learn to talk.

I was glad I had Jeremy's name on the list for a workshop through the Wisconsin clinic. No one except Randall seemed to understand why I felt Jeremy wasn't getting enough out of the special ed class. It felt like the whole world was against us.

***

Jeremy's teacher had signed me up for a seminar on autism in Waco. On the way there, I thought about how removing foods Jeremy was allergic to, eliminating processed meat from his diet, and giving him vitamins seemed to help him. He no longer had that wild-eyed look, and he was beginning to get some language back. Slowly Randall and I had found some of the pieces of the puzzle that uniquely fit Jeremy's needs, but we had a long way to go.

Arriving about five minutes early for the seminar, I sat down at a table with some other women awaiting the speaker. After we had introduced ourselves, I found that I was the only parent in the group. All the rest were teachers. One lady looked completely bored. A couple of others talked about how much this seminar would count toward some sort of continuing education requirements.

An attractive young teacher next to me said, "What school district do you teach in?"

"Actually, I'm a parent." I went on to explain Jeremy's diagnosis and my search for help.

"Wow, I wouldn't be surprised if your son becomes President someday." The remark came with a smile. Searching her face to discover if she was being sarcastic, I found only sincerity. The compliment warmed me.

While we discussed Jeremy's situation, the speaker for the day walked up to the front, ready to begin. He introduced himself as Harry Jones (not his real name) from North Carolina. He worked with a group from the University of North Carolina called TEACCH (The Treatment and Education of Autistic and related Communication-handicapped CHildren). "I'd like to begin the day with a film."

Between the film Mr. Jones showed us and his speech, I gained a new realization of the difficulties autistic people and their families experience. One autistic man would stop and put his mouth on street signs as he walked down the road. Another man washed dishes for a restaurant in his hometown. When something out of the ordinary happened, he would start screaming. Since he couldn't talk, it was difficult to understand how to help him. A young woman worked in a factory and had a productive job. However, at break time she would beat her head against the wall. Obviously, her co-workers found it disconcerting, so the TEACCH caseworker told her to find someplace else to have her breaks.

Behaviors such as head banging, rocking, spinning the body, gazing at lights, clicking the tongue, fixation on rotating objects, and flapping hands are prevalent in autistic individuals. Such behavior is called self-stimulation.

As the disabled individuals lived out their lives on the screen, the images shocked me. My heart plummeted. *I thought I knew what autism was.* My reading had not prepared me for its realities.

The speaker seemed proud of some of the cases in the film. Apparently, from his perspective, many of these autistic individuals had reached some level of success. The autistic adults on the film did work and had some productivity, but this wasn't enough for me. I had higher hopes for Jeremy's future. After the film, Mr. Jones dismissed us for a short break before continuing his presentation.

Since my table was close to the podium, I took the opportunity to introduce myself to Mr. Jones. After exchanging pleasantries and filling him in on some of Jeremy's background, I said, "We've got our name on a waiting list for a consultant to come and teach us how to do the therapy started by Dr. Lovaas of UCLA. I've watched a film where Dr. Lovaas and his colleagues revealed a study they had conducted of 19 children where 9 of the kids were able to reach normal functioning. Don't you think I should try this therapy approach first since some of the kids in the study have grown up to live normal lives?"

"Well, I—"

A woman interrupted, "It's time to start again, everyone."

"Excuse me," he said.

The start of the session went right to the issue I had just brought up.

"The treatments available for autism vary. One approach is what I call conquering autism." He didn't say it, but I knew he was talking about ABA therapy. "It requires 30 to 40 hours of one-on-one per week, and it does make recovery possible in some cases. This approach is too costly for school systems. A small percentage of autistic individuals can't be helped by TEACCH or any of the other approaches for that matter." Mr. Jones glanced at me during this part of his speech. The words didn't come across as someone advocating a possible cure, even though technically he said you could "conquer" autism. Instead of sounding optimistic, he conveyed skepticism for any therapy approach that could be perceived as a cure. His tone of voice contradicted the words and communicated a completely different meaning.

*Why wouldn't I want to do this if there is a possibility of recovery? What's wrong with conquering autism? Why wouldn't I want my son to avoid the kind of lives depicted in the film?* I wanted to say something out loud, but politeness kept me silent.

*Why does he talk like conquering autism is such a ridiculous thing?* I didn't understand. I wondered if my face revealed how baffled I felt.

Dragging my thoughts back to the speaker, I heard him say some of the assumptions TEACCH had made about autism: "Their nervous systems cannot process information, and they cannot learn as we do. When we work with autistic individuals, we take into account the child or adult's deficits and structure their lives so they can handle the classroom or workplace. Structure is the key to making life bearable for them."

I stayed for the two-day seminar and left with a notebook of information, eight pages of notes, and a respect for this group.

Driving home, my thoughts ran ninety miles an hour. If Jeremy doesn't make it with the ABA therapy, we'll try TEACCH. It takes into account all the deficits and idiosyncrasies of autism. However, I hoped we wouldn't need TEACCH. Autism and special needs was a whole world that I didn't know existed until a few months ago, and I didn't want my son or our family to have to live in that world if I could prevent it.

Why didn't the ABA people and TEACCH work together more? They both had so much to contribute to the field. As a parent I didn't care who helped Jeremy the most, I just wanted results. Time was ticking away. I wanted action.

# CHAPTER EIGHT:
# PROCRASTINATORS, VITAMINS,
# AND JENNIFER'S SOLUTION

Randall and I had to be among the world's worst procrastinators. Knowing us, we would discuss having a workshop for weeks, months, years until one day Jeremy would be six. If we were to provide meaningful help for Jeremy, procrastinating was not an option.

I began daily work sessions with Jeremy while I ignored everyone and everything except him. Sometimes Randall helped me. Our work sessions lacked the correct therapy approach, but I couldn't stand watching Jeremy do nothing all day long. He seemed to be losing ground every minute. I set up a child-size table and chairs in Jeremy's room. After several trips to the educational store I purchased some materials to help us.

I sat on the floor watching Randall work with Jeremy. Determination showed in every muscle on Randall's face as he began to teach some action verbs to Jeremy, pressing Jeremy as hard as he could within reason. Randall focused on the session like it would cure everything, and Jeremy resisted with all his might.

"If Jeremy could just get through learning his verbs…" Randall said, leaving his sentence hanging with implied meaning. Then he brought Jeremy back to the table.

"What is he doing?" Randall asked Jeremy as he pointed to a picture of a man drinking. "Say 'drinking'."

Jeremy cried and put his head on the table.

Randall persisted. Raising his voice, he said, "What is he doing? Say 'drinking'."

I sensed Randall's frustration and feared he was about to lose his temper.

Unfocused and uncooperative, Jeremy hung his head upside down while letting his bottom stay in the chair.

"At least he stopped crying. Uh, I think we are doing something wrong, Randall. We're supposed to make this fun and rewarding." I softened my voice so I wouldn't add to the tense atmosphere that filled the room.

Knowing it could easily be me who was frustrated, I remained quiet. I understood firsthand how frustrating it was to teach Jeremy. Why were autistic kids so resistant to learning?

Continuing as if Jeremy's life depended on it, Randall worked on verbs until Jeremy could identify and say three verbs. The work session resembled a game of tug-of-war, and I wasn't sure who had won this round. If an ABA consultant had been watching, I'm sure she would have cringed. We needed help badly.

"Okay, Jeremy, you can go have a snack," Randall said through gritted teeth.

The set of Randall's jaw told of the strain of the work session.

"Why does he resist so much?" Randall questioned—aggravation evident in every word.

"I get put out with him, too. It feels like swimming in mud trying to teach him anything. It's hard to keep my cool when I think he should cooperate." I sat cross-legged and put my hands on my knees. "You know? We get the idea if we can just get him to learn verbs, or this, or that, or whatever it is at the moment, everything would be all right, and he would start making progress with his learning."

Randall nodded. Sad eyes met mine. He jerked his fingers through his hair over and over, frustration apparent in every movement.

My mind rushed to come up with a way to explain what I needed to get across. "He's not much better off now than he was before the three verbs. I think a good analogy is like taking a lost child through a forest. You have to go all the way to the other side with him and make sure he is safe. You can't say, 'He's made it the first mile through the forest, so therefore, he can make it all the way by himself.' No, you have to help him the whole way."

"Yeah, I…"

"Oh, no!" I glanced at my watch. "I need to go pick up Jennifer at school."

"Yeah, I have to get back to work anyway."

Picking up my keys, I loaded Jeremy in the car and headed for the school.

Jennifer jumped in the car, giving me a big smile. "Hi, Mommy. Hi, Jeremy."

Jeremy stared out the window.

"Mommy, I want Jeremy to play with me when we get home. Why doesn't Jeremy ever play with me?" Jennifer asked, but she didn't stop for an answer. "You know what I did today, Mommy. I asked my teacher if we could pray for Jeremy because he isn't talking."

"Good, honey, thank you." Jennifer attended a Christian school, and I knew the kids started their day with prayer. *What a sweet little girl I have!* "What did you do in school today?"

Before Jennifer could answer, a mother of one of Jennifer's classmates waved me down, so I pulled over and rolled down my window.

"I know this is late notice," she said, "but could Jennifer come over and play with Emily right now? I can bring her home in about an hour."

*Oh, good, Jennifer needs some fun.* "Sure, that'll be great. She'll be glad for something to do. But why don't I pick her up? Jeremy has an appointment right now, and we could pick her up on the way home."

"Yea!" Jennifer leaped out the car and headed toward Emily. They chattered and laughed their way to an Explorer parked a few feet away.

"Thanks, Karen."

"Sure, thank you for asking."

I guided the car out of the parking lot, glancing at my cute little boy in his car seat. "We have just enough time to get to your speech therapy session, Jeremy."

A few minutes later, Joan, who had been Jeremy's speech therapist since he had turned three, greeted us and led us to her office. Watching the therapy, I hung on to every word, hoping and praying for progress. It seemed impossible to measure growth. Was the aim random language?

At the end of the hour I handed her payment for recent sessions. "Did you read *Let Me Hear Your Voice* I gave you about the autistic child who after intense therapy made it to normal functioning?" I asked her.

"Yes," she responded, reaching inside a drawer and handing me the book. "The curriculum in the back of the book is fantastic. I've never seen better."

"This is what I want to do for Jeremy. But I'm not getting very much support from the public school professionals."

"Go for it, Karen." Joan gave me an encouraging smile. "It sounds good."

I felt enormous relief. I had never realized until this struggle started how much others' approval really meant to me. It helped to have someone support me in this endeavor to help Jeremy, even if it was only verbal encouragement. Some days even Randall didn't seem convinced we should use the Wisconsin clinic and implement an ABA therapy program. Support from my husband, parents, sisters, and friends was important to me. However, the stakes were too high to wait for everyone's approval. I had to do the right thing now, regardless. I didn't have time to wait much longer.

I now knew two professionals who had encouraged me to go ahead with the therapy: Joan and a psychologist who attended the autism support group. Not good odds—two professionals against the world. It might sound as if I was exaggerating, but in my world this was the probability.

Later, Linda, the friend from the autism parent support group, called me at home. "Karen," she said. "I've got some of that Super Nu-Thera multi-vitamin powder for autistic children. It turns out that George is allergic to it. Would you like to have it?"

"Yes, Jeremy's been taking it, and I think it's helping. But let me pay you for it." Holding the kitchen phone between my chin and my shoulder, I opened the refrigerator to see what I could cook for dinner. I could hear Jennifer in the living room trying to get Jeremy to play with her. Her efforts met with his usual lack of interest.

"No, I want to give you the powder. It will go to waste if you don't use it."

"Thank you, that is sweet of you."

"My mother is going to drop it off when she runs errands tomorrow after school. Will you be home?"

"Yeah, thanks, Linda."

I went back to planning dinner. *Should I have a short cut meal of baked potatoes or make pizza from scratch?* Jeremy loved pizza. I made pizza from scratch because of his allergies. If I cooked it myself, I knew what was in it.

Opening the small drawer in the refrigerator, I found pizza cheese. *Good. I guess I'm making pizza.* The sound of *Captain Planet* on the living room TV drifted into the kitchen. I wasn't sure I liked Jeremy watching Captain Planet. He got off on some of the words and would echo them later. Even though I wanted him to talk, the rare language of Captain Planet words echoed at unexpected times wasn't good. A commercial came on, and I could hear Jennifer insisting, "Let's play a game, Jeremy."

"No." Jeremy seemed to pry the word out with a great effort. My heart sunk. His language came so hard.

Poor Jennifer. *I'm going to have to explain to her what's going on.* I wasn't sure what a seven-year-old could understand, but I needed to try. Jeremy received so much more attention these days. I wonder if I can explain that to her, too.

I kneaded the pizza dough and then pounded it with my fist.

*Tomorrow, I need to get Jeremy tested for the Wisconsin clinic requirements before starting the workshops. Maybe the public school would do it for me.* I had told the teacher I would be pulling Jeremy out of school to do therapy thirty-six hours a week. It just wasn't practical to try to keep both school and therapy going. As far as I could tell, the teacher had taken my news well, so I had high hopes she would help me with the testing.

My dad didn't like the idea of working Jeremy thirty-six to forty hours a week. I respected my dad, but I knew the intensive therapy was the right thing to do. *I'm an adult now. It's time to follow my own convictions.* I hoped once we learned the correct methods Jeremy would be able to tolerate the hours. *Therapy is bound to be better than having him sit in front of the TV all day flapping his hands.*

An unusual silence came from the living room. Jennifer must have given up trying to get Jeremy to interact with her. The timer went off, and as I turned to reach for the oven mittens, Jennifer walked in the kitchen. To my surprise and amusement she had a rope tied around her waist. On the other end of the rope she had tied Jeremy. He obediently followed her around, the rope dangling between them about two feet.

"Come on, Jeremy," Jennifer said, leading him in circles from the living room and then back into the kitchen.

I'm not sure what amused me the most, Jennifer's interesting solution to the problem of getting Jeremy to relate to her, or Jeremy docilely following her around.

Having a good laugh for the first time in a while, I called everyone in to eat pizza.

# CHAPTER NINE:
# GET READY, GET SET . . .

The sound of the doorbell reverberated through the house. Walking to the door, I looked through the peephole and saw Linda's mother with the vitamins for Jeremy, along with George, Linda's 9-year-old autistic son.

Opening the door, I greeted her. "Hi, thank you for coming, Mrs. Carson. Come on in for a little while and visit."

Mrs. Carson and George came in. George proceeded to hit the walls with his hands, one of his self-stimulation behaviors. I had only met George twice before. Both times he kept up constant stimming motions. Stimming is short for self-stimulation behaviors such at head banging, rocking, spinning the body, gazing at lights, or flapping hands. All are common behaviors in autistic individuals.

"Did you know we didn't know George was autistic until he was six years old?" Mrs. Carson asked. "Then the doctor finally gave us a diagnosis. When he was three, he used to talk and interact with people. Then he began to lose language and…" She let her words drift off, her lips in a straight line and her brows pushed together. "I wish the doctor had told us sooner."

As far as I could tell George didn't hear our conversation. He continued banging on the walls, moving from one wall to the next. Jeremy walked by and looked up at George. *Since when was Jeremy interested in anyone?* For Jeremy this was progress. Perhaps throwing all the intervention at Jeremy had begun to pay off. We had made a good start. Jeremy's stimming behaviors had decreased, and I was starting to hear some language again. I wondered how the testing would come out. The public school had consented to do the testing, except for the IQ test.

Mrs. Carson glanced from me to George, then down at Jeremy. "How do you know anything is wrong? He doesn't look autistic to me."

I sighed and gave her a grim smile. "Mainly Jeremy's history. If you only knew…"

"I'm glad you found out when he was so young. I think it makes a big difference." She glanced at her watch. "Oh, I've got to get going." Starting toward the door, she turned to George. "Come on, George. We need to go."

George had no trouble following these instructions. He made a couple of pats on the wall and walked out the front door. Amazed, I thanked her and closed the door. Maybe George understood people's language more than I thought.

\*\*\*

After playing phone tag with the speech therapist at Jeremy's school, we finally were able to agree on a time that I could pick up Jeremy's test results. She was working at another campus several blocks away from Jeremy's school. So I picked up Jeremy after his special ed preschool class and drove to the other campus.

Handing over the envelope with Jeremy's test papers, she said, "It is possible Jeremy is doing better than this test reflects, but we're not allowed to help him along during the test."

"I understand." I opened the envelope and looked at the score. I needed privacy to absorb this. So I cut our conversation short and gave her what I hoped was a gracious "thank you" and hurried home to mull over the test results.

At home, I dropped my purse and the large envelope on the table, gave Jeremy a snack, and then pulled the test results out of the envelope.

Hoping for a miracle, I scanned the results. No matter how I read the outcome, Jeremy was still developmentally about two years behind his current age of three years and four months.

Although we had worked hard and spent hours giving Jeremy attention, our efforts hadn't measured up to what he needed.

I remembered talking to other mothers of autistic kids who had spent many hours with their children. Though their children had made significant strides under the circumstances, none had succeeded in overcoming autism. Their children still had many issues they had never been able to deal with. Why should I be surprised? *Remember the words in the material on autism— lifelong, incapacitating, incurable.*

All the hard work we had put into Jeremy's therapy so far seemed to have had little impact. I thought of all the hours teaching verbs, labeling items, and playing games with him.

I felt as if he was doing better, even though the test didn't reflect it. Whatever the level of improvement, he still couldn't interact with other children his age or talk at his age level. He needed intense one-on-one therapy. I thought of my analogy of taking a lost child safely through a forest. Jeremy hadn't arrived safely home, therefore, we would continue with plans for intense therapy.

In the eight months since his last test, his communication skills had progressed developmentally from six months to eighteen months, and his socialization had progressed from ten months old to nineteen months old. Though it was an improvement, he was still considerably behind his peers.

\*\*\*

The Wisconsin clinic required still more testing, so Jeremy and I made the 120-mile trip to College Station, Texas, to visit an old friend of mine from high school, psychologist Dr. Roy Luepnitz, PhD. He had promised to do the last of the testing needed for the Wisconsin clinic. After a nice visit with Roy and his wife, I followed Roy in our car to his counseling office.

"You and Jeremy can wait here in the playroom. I'll get everything set up, Karen."

"Thanks."

Roy left, and I sat down to watch Jeremy play. The office was silent except for the clicking of the receptionist's keyboard in the next room. Roy had graciously cleared his schedule to focus on Jeremy.

The playroom provided children with all kinds of toys—a miniature basketball goal in the corner, puzzles, books—everything imaginable. "Jeremy, do this puzzle."

Without resistance, Jeremy began to work the puzzle. He loved puzzles. I was glad. If I could only fill his whole day with working puzzles, I wouldn't have any problems.

Roy came to the door. "I'm ready for Jeremy now."

I stood and took Jeremy's hand, and we followed Roy to a nearby office.

Knowing I was not allowed to prompt or help Jeremy with the test, I kept quiet. I watched Roy try to engage Jeremy in answering questions, but Jeremy didn't know the answers. Then Roy tried asking a question from a different section of the test book. Still Jeremy couldn't answer. Roy made more attempts, but soon shut the test book and placed it in a box.

Looking over at me, Roy said, "He can't be tested. He just isn't developmentally ready for this test. Take Jeremy to the playroom, and I'll write up something for you to give the Wisconsin clinic."

I twirled a strand of hair and bit my lower lip. "Thanks."

Shortly afterwards, Roy came in and handed me some paperwork. He glanced over at Jeremy and then looked back at me. "Jeremy is behaving too well to be diagnosed with autism. I consider him to have a severe receptive/expressive language delay."

Though saying Jeremy had a severe receptive/expressive language delay rather than autism should have comforted me, I felt amazingly void of any emotions good or bad. After weeks of research and applying what we'd learned, I felt this less acute diagnosis only meant we had had some effect. To some parents of autistic kids this diagnosis could be interpreted to mean their children didn't need more work. I knew better than that. I had seen other parents accept a level of achievement from a child when more work could have helped him/her learn and grow into a more productive person. In most cases, parents seemed to go into denial and develop false hopes of their children having complete recovery.

Jeremy needed to learn what other preschool children knew, his language needed so much help, and he needed to learn social skills. He was developmentally two years behind the standard for his age and didn't interact with his peers. This all translated into more work for us. We were on the right road—we just needed to persevere.

***

The following week I began interviewing people to work with Jeremy. I went to a local university employment office that provided jobs for students. In the job description I tried to appeal to idealistic college students and placed the hourly rate a little higher than that paid by the local fast food restaurants.

I called a local home school number. When a woman answered, I asked if she knew anyone who had older children willing to work. She gave me a phone number. Anxious to get going with Jeremy's therapy, I immediately called and talked to a homeschooler who had three older sons.

"Here, you can talk to my oldest son, Zack. He has graduated from college and works as a tutor for several children right now."

His qualifications sounded wonderful.

"Hello." The voice of a young man spoke over the phone line.

I introduced myself to Zack. I appealed to the young man and fervently spoke up for Jeremy's cause. I explained what we were doing for Jeremy. I must have been effective because Zack said he would come and interview for the job. He said he had plenty of work hours but felt working with Jeremy would be a good experience for him. *Wonderful. I'm glad he's not worried about the money, because I can't pay very much.*

I was excited about this step in the right direction. It felt good to get started.

During the next few days I hired Zack and interviewed several other young people. Needing to fill at least five positions, I changed my ad to read, "Tutor needed" instead of "Therapist needed."

The students who had responded to my ad communicated that they didn't feel qualified to be therapists and therefore had hesitated to call. Since I could provide the training, there was nothing to worry about. I needed a tutor kind of person. So I made new flyers, but this time I placed them on the walls of the local Christian university and a local community college, trying to interest special education majors and psychology majors.

One young woman I hired quit after two weeks. Her leaving pained me so much I decided to ask in the interviews for a six-month commitment. One blessing came from the bad experience—I found three other girls through the girl who quit. Maybe that's what God had intended all along.

The call finally came for scheduling the first workshop. Crystal, who had done Kayla's workshop in Austin, called. "I can do a workshop in January. How about the weekend after New Year's Day?"

The question sent an immediate burst of adrenalin coursing through me. Whew! The weeks of waiting had paid off. We had a workshop set for January.

"Yes!" I said.

# CHAPTER TEN:

# GO... YES! THE FIRST ABA WORKSHOP!

I called my sister, Liz, to share with her my excitement at having scheduled our first workshop. "Liz, guess what? We have a three-day workshop scheduled for Jeremy. I'm so excited. I think this is really going to help us."

"Now, explain to me how this works, Karen. Is this just for Jeremy? And who attends?"

"It's a workshop just for Jeremy—with only our therapists, Randall, and me. We're paying for a workshop fee and travel expenses for the consultant. Then I pay the hourly rate for our therapists' time. Of course, I have to feed everyone, too. We'll need to do this every two or three months. But after this first workshop, all the others will be two days long. Each day we will work in the morning, break for lunch, and then have an afternoon session."

"Wow, this is really something. I'm glad you're getting help."

"Years ago I remember wondering what it would take to rescue someone who had a severe problem. Now I think it takes a team, a mega effort that most people don't even think about. They consider twenty minutes of therapy a day adequate in helping a child with a disability like Jeremy's. Normal kids are learning every waking moment, so scheduling forty hours will give Jeremy more of a fighting chance. We want to stimulate learning and exercise his brain."

"You know, I was telling my mother-in-law this week about how hard you've been working and how much progress Jeremy has made since you removed the food he is allergic to and started giving him those vitamins that are high in B6 and Magnesium. She was so touched she cried. She told me to tell you to keep it up."

Hearing Mrs. Richardson's words moved me. I had been praying the Lord would send me some encouragement. *The Lord is so good.* He had answered my prayer. I hadn't expected to get the message through Mrs. Richardson, who lived in West Virginia.

"Are you still there, Karen?"

"Yes, I'm sorry. I'm crying." My voice quivered as I spoke. "I'd been praying for some encouragement, and the Lord sent it to me." The tears continued rolling down my cheeks.

"I'll tell Mrs. Richardson you said that, Karen," she said, with a smile in her voice.

We said our goodbyes, and I marveled at the timing of this conversation. The Lord had heard my prayers. I just needed to be patient.

In the days leading up to the first workshop I busied myself with all the preparations needed. I wanted the therapists to know as much as possible so that we could use our time wisely. Why not use every minute of the three-day workshop?

I had hoped other children's workshops would have helped us with teaching Jeremy, but I discovered that though the principles were the same, the program needed to be tailored for each child's needs.

The five young people I hired had already started working with Jeremy before our consultant, Crystal, came for the first workshop. We had worked with Jeremy on drills such as matching, simple one-step commands, prepositions, and other beginning principles.

Though Jeremy was learning under our amateur attempts, we lacked the techniques we needed. I hoped our attempts hadn't been a complete disaster. I had heard horror stories of parents who tried the therapy without help only to make mistakes that caused difficulty in working with their child later. Some days Jeremy enjoyed working and learning from us—at other times he didn't. Even though we had taken a stab at tracking Jeremy's progress, we had no good way of documenting what we did. We needed a way to pass information and progress from one therapist to the next person. I feared the work sessions with Jeremy had turned into hit-and-miss teaching times. We needed to introduce new drills, but I had no idea what kind. Most importantly, Jeremy lacked compliance. We needed help.

Maybe I should have waited for the first workshop to begin working, but, no, that thought was unacceptable.

*Too fearful—that's what my problem is.* Any waiting period before beginning to help Jeremy felt too long.

Scheduling the workshop during the Christmas break had caused problems—only Zack and Heather could come. Randall suggested that I reschedule, but I couldn't bear it. *Maybe I should put the matter in God's hands and reschedule.* I didn't know. I told Randall, "I'm too concerned for Jeremy to put this off. I'm not waiting another minute."

On the drive to the Austin airport to pick up Crystal for the first workshop, I thought about the work sessions we had had with Jeremy since hiring extra help. A few days earlier, I had filmed Heather working with Jeremy and had mailed the video to Crystal so she could get an idea on how the program had progressed.

For one drill, Heather placed ten pictures out on the table of simple objects such as pig, dog, tree, ladder, banana, etc. Then she handed Jeremy a picture of a pig. "Jeremy, put with same."

Jeremy smiled and placed the pig on top of the other pig. He enjoyed it.

"Good job, Jeremy." Heather continued handing him cards and making the same request until he correctly responded by matching all the pictures.

To see Jeremy do productive activities felt good.

For the next drill Heather pulled out a big stuffed turtle and placed it on the table. "Where is the turtle?"

"On," Jeremy answered in a high-pitched voice, his articulation so poor it was hard to decipher if he had said the right word. Heather continued placing the turtle in various places until he identified "under" and "beside." With a basket on top of the table, she illustrated "in." When she started working on "behind" by placing the turtle behind her back, Jeremy got up and walked off. He picked up his 101 Dalmatian pillow and laid down on it. Clearly he didn't plan to work any longer. How should we handle this? Should we just let him go or what?

Were we working him too long? Did we have the correct technique? Were we making learning clear and concise for him? How could we get better compliance? All these questions I hoped Crystal could answer.

At the terminal I searched the crowd for the blonde young woman. I caught sight of her exiting the gate area.

"Crystal." I waved my hand to get her attention.

She recognized me from our introduction at Kayla's workshop and greeted me.

"Did you check any luggage?" I glanced down at a large carry-on bag and gave her an inquiring look.

"No, this is it."

After getting on the road, we began to discuss Jeremy and therapy. Hearing about Crystal's experiences with her other patients helped. I absorbed every piece of information she offered. She was a fountain of information, so I began to ask questions.

"How many families do you work with?"

"Besides a few local children, I have fifteen families from out of state—from New York to Alabama, then some families in Illinois and Michigan. Just the eastern part of the United States. The west coast—the UCLA clinic handles. I do weekend workshops twice a month. I work with a wide range of children—from children who aren't talking to children who are being mainstreamed into kindergarten."

"Are y'all having the same success rate as the UCLA study?"

"Actually, we are. Since the clinic opened, we have gotten the same results as UCLA."

That was good. I still didn't know if Jeremy would be among the children who reached normalcy, but at least I knew I had a knowledgeable clinic involved in helping us.

"What else do you want to talk about?" she asked.

I smiled at her. "Everything." And until we got home I kept her talking.

During the first hours of the workshop, Crystal worked with me and began evaluating Jeremy's skills before bringing in anyone else to work. As we talked that first day, Jeremy sat contentedly with his toys in the same room while Crystal and I discussed therapy issues. Most children would need a babysitter or some entertainment to occupy their time, but Jeremy still was not sociable. He seemed content to be alone for hours at a time unless we sought him out. I hoped one day we would need to hire a babysitter during workshops while the therapist, Randall, and I worked.

"Crystal, Jeremy's lining up toys. That's something we need to stop, right?" I had read that many autistic children and adults have an obsessive habit of lining up their favorite objects, and I wondered what to do about it.

Reaching over the notes in her hand, she rearranged the toys in a different way. "Yes, change the position of the toys every time you see him lining up objects."

Later in the workshop the first group session took place with Randall, Zack, Heather, and me in attendance. Crystal told us about the clinic, the therapy, and her qualifications. "Dr. Lovaas, along with his researchers, thought if language was taught to autistic children that other behavior would automatically come. But this wasn't true. Play skills were still minimal. The children still needed help learning to interact with others, developing play skills, participating in non-verbal activities, etc. In other words, everything has to be taught."

Crystal turned a page in her notebook. "Jeremy will need to have around forty hours of therapy per week. Then when he is ready for preschool, we will need to phase in school hours and phase out therapy hours. In addition, he will need peer play, which will also increase as the therapy hours decrease."

"How many hours are we going to do?" Heather asked.

Everyone looked at me for the answer.

I glanced at Heather. She sat on our couch leaning her arm on the armrest, brown hair hitting shoulder-length, her petite-frame dressed neatly but casually in a pair of fashionable jeans and knit top. Heather hadn't worked for me long, but I was pleased with her efforts. She had a love and commitment to Jeremy that any mother would value. Heather was conscientious and had made a sacrifice to come to the workshop. The university she attended didn't resume classes until the following week, but she had made the trip all the way from the Texas coast to be at the workshop.

I responded to Heather's question. "At this point, I'm scheduling 36 hours, six hours, six days a week. I'm not going to schedule Sunday unless it's a workshop. If someone really wants to make up some hours, I'll let them work a Sunday afternoon." I felt we needed a day to rest and just go to church without worrying about a schedule. At the same time I didn't want to be legalistic and unmovable, so I was open to exceptions. "If 36 hours is not enough, I can increase the hours later. We still have to work around Jeremy's naps. He still takes a nap right after lunch."

While we talked, Jeremy kept up a nonsensical chatter from the next room, I wondered if this babbling meant anything? Maybe we had stimulated his brain enough to cause him to go through the developmental stage that babies are in when they babble. I hoped his chatter was a precursor to talking. Maybe he was speaking words already but just couldn't articulate the words distinctly enough to be understood. Whatever the chatter meant, it sounded good.

Crystal glanced down at her notes. "The whole theory behind this program is operant conditioning, meaning every behavior has a consequence. In other words, consequences affect behavior. We want to increase positive reinforcements for every correct response. We'll start easy so that we can teach that learning is rewarding." Crystal glanced at each of us, placed her elbow on her knees, chin in her hands. "What else would you like to talk about before we call Jeremy to the table and work on drills?"

Randall spoke up. "Karen has been afraid Jeremy won't show affection or form attachments to people. But I think he's getting better."

"Great. That certainly is one of the goals."

Crystal straightened her paperwork and continued. "We use a discrete trial format. You issue a command, instruction, or question. After the child responds to that command, you reward him or give an informational 'no' for wrong responses or a lack of response. It's important to be clear and concise." Picking up some papers, she handed one to me. "Here is a handout for the meaning of discrete trail format and some other therapy terms."

"We're having a lot of problems holding Jeremy's attention much less making instructions clear and concise," Randall said.

"I'm not sure we have found the best rewards for him." I pointed out.

Crystal pushed a strand of blonde hair behind her ear. "As you work with him, come up with a list of rewards he enjoys. Things such as bubbles, balloons, noisemakers, or verbal praise are some ideas. Crazy therapists usually make the best therapists." She smiled. "If we are entertained watching someone work with the child, then the child is entertained."

Jeremy ran through the living room with Jennifer right behind him then disappeared from my view.

My gaze jumped back to Crystal. Looking down at her notes, she turned a page. "Sometimes parents question a drill being introduced because their child knows the information to be practiced. The child needs to learn compliance as well as knowledge in order to be successful in the classroom. If a teacher asks something of a child and he knows it, but is not compliant enough to answer, then knowing the information is not enough."

"How do we work on play skills?" Zach questioned.

"You teach each play activity independently, and after Jeremy has enough appropriate play skills you set up play stations in the room, such as Legos, Superman, etc. You start playing at a play station. Hopefully, he comes and plays. If not, you prompt him. Eventually, you work up to ten play stations. I'll explain more when he is ready."

Jennifer and Jeremy ran past us again, settling back in the playroom just off the living room.

After our discussion session, Crystal announced we would work with Jeremy at the table with drills. I had been looking forward to this part of the workshop. We had been learning in theory up until now. I was ready for some hands-on training.

"Karen, you start by doing the *Block Imitation* drill with Jeremy."

# CHAPTER ELEVEN:

# LET'S GET DOWN TO BUSINESS

I stood up to do the block drill with Jeremy, drawing in a deep breath as I attempted to relax. An ache formed in my chest. I glanced around the room at Randall, Heather, Zach, and Crystal.

All right, here goes—my turn to teach Jeremy one of the drills Crystal had assigned us to teach him. Why should something so simple to execute feel so important to me?

Though we had taught Jeremy many beginning principles before the workshop started, we still had some beginning drills in his program, such as *Receptive Commands* and *Nonverbal Imitation* on the list. In these two drills we taught easy instructions such as stand up, sit down, clap hands, stomp feet, etc. I was bored to tears teaching these things. I knew Jeremy needed to learn to follow basic instructions and to be compliant, but it was hard to be patient.

How could Jeremy go on to more difficult instructions unless he could comply with easy directions? I wanted to think Jeremy was ready for more advanced drills, but I knew Jeremy needed drills like these as first steps toward the more advanced concepts.

"Okay. I'm doing the *Block Imitation* drill, right?"

Crystal nodded.

I walked over and set the blocks on the table to get ready for the drill. I pulled out six wood blocks of different shapes and colors and made a random pattern that Jeremy needed to imitate.

Then I laid out matching blocks on his side of the table. Crystal and I had already figured out he could imitate a pattern of five without help, so we began with a six-block pattern to challenge him. It seemed like a great brain exercise for him.

I went to get Jeremy, who was sitting on the floor in the playroom with toys tossed around him. My heart filled with love for him. He looked so cute in his sweat suit with the stripe down the side of the arms and legs. Walking Jeremy into the living room where we were holding the workshop, I guided him to sit down. He cooperated.

Before I started the drill, I mumbled, "Make Mommy look good." Heather and Zack laughed. I pointed to my blocks. "Do this."

We had spent hours with Jeremy teaching labeling, colors, matching, and more. And we had many more hours to go. Every piece of information we taught him brought us closer to the goal. I wanted Crystal to give us drills right on the cutting edge of his learning ability.

I smiled as Jeremy reached for a block. To encourage him to keep working, I urged him on with an occasional, "Good ... Right."

Jeremy took a few seconds, but he successfully placed his blocks in the same pattern.

We all burst into applause. Jeremy appeared shocked at the attention but then broke into a wide grin.

I beamed. "Good, Jeremy. Go play."

As Jeremy ran into the next room, Crystal said, "*Block imitation* helps build a longer attention span. I'm leaving an instruction sheet on how to progress with this drill."

"How long should we work when we call him to the table? Do we work him the whole two hours when I schedule a time slot?"

"For every 45 minutes, there's a 15 minute break. That counts for an hour."

I mentally filed that information in my mind and came up with another question. "How long do we keep him at the table each time?"

"For most drills about five to seven requests or commands. Then he gets a break for a minute or so while you get ready for the next drill."

This information was comforting. Even a three-year-old could handle that schedule. It didn't seem too harsh to me. Calling Jeremy to the table would draw him from the world he had withdrawn to and teach him appropriate skills at the same time. The thought gave me some peace in the midst of my intense focus to learn all I needed to make this therapy work for Jeremy.

Zach taught *Nonverbal Imitation* for his turn.

*Boring. I'm glad I didn't get this drill.*

Zach called Jeremy back to the table, but Jeremy began to cry. Taking a no-nonsense approach, Zach calmly walked over to Jeremy, gently picked him up, and put him on the chair. This caused a full-blown tantrum, which happened all too often. These tantrums were one of the main reasons we needed professional help. Zach and everyone in the room appeared unaffected by the tantrum. Part of handling bad behavior was to ignore it. If we responded to the tantrum and gave in to it, Jeremy would learn he only had to cry to get out of working.

Jeremy twisted his body and fell on the floor. His crying escalated.

Zach reached down, and patiently situated him back on the chair. Though Jeremy continued to cry, Zach illustrated clapping hands and said, "Do this."

Wiggling around on the seat, crying at high volume, Jeremy nevertheless clapped his own hands.

We applauded and yelled out from our places. "Good. That's right!"

Surprised out of his tantrum, Jeremy stopped crying. After Zach did about four more commands and reinforced correct responses, Zach gave an upbeat, "Go play."

Jeremy left the table happy and went back to the playroom.

"See?" Crystal affirmed. "When you work through the tantrum he learns it didn't help to cry. If you give in to the crying, you reinforce the tantrum. If everyone in his life ignores tantrums, the tantrums should decline and eventually disappear. Also, you need to end the drill in success."

"What if you can't get him to respond? How can you end in success if that happens?" I asked. I had found out it's easier to say "end a drill in success," than to accomplish it.

"Sometimes you have to prompt success. For instance, if you ask him to clap his hands, and he won't, pick up his hands and clap for him. Reinforce as if he complied and tell him to go play."

"Okay, thanks, that sounds worth a try."

I glanced into the playroom. Jeremy sat playing with some plastic sea creatures. He appeared unaware that we had talked about him for hours, oblivious to the fact that working with him for hours was unique to a three year old. Would the average three year old ask why all these people were here, and why they were working with him?

Next Heather called Jeremy to the table for the *What's Missing* drill. Heather placed three items and a box lid on the table. When Jeremy sat down at the table, she pointed to each item one at a time going from left to right. "Car ... Cup ... Baby." Then she placed the box lid in front of the items, blocking Jeremy's view. She reached behind the box lid and removed the cup and then the box lid.

Now, all the items were in view except for the cup. She looked at Jeremy. "What's missing?"

"Cup," Jeremy responded in a high-pitched voice. Some day we would need to address a way to correct Jeremy's voice tone and pitch, but for now we had all we could handle.

Heather repeated the "what's missing" question a few times, using various items and randomly selecting a different missing item each time. "Great working, Jeremy. Go play."

"Why don't you go ahead and do the *Emotion* drill, Heather?" I suggested.

Calling Jeremy back to the work chair, Heather acted like she was afraid and exclaimed, "How do I feel? Say 'scared'."

"Cad." Jeremy's articulation was so bad I wasn't sure he got the right answer. The word came out nothing like the word *scared*.

Heather didn't seem to know how to react either. She must have believed he had the right answer because she reluctantly responded, "Good, Jeremy," cutting a quick glance at Crystal.

We all began to talk at once. Randall asked Jeremy to say the word *scared*. Someone else asked him to say the word *afraid*. Crystal told us to practice words Jeremy had a hard time pronouncing during the *Verbal Imitation* drill.

"I want to try again," Heather stated, glancing quickly from us back to Jeremy.

Heather's hands flew to her mouth in a defensive posture and repeated, "How do I feel?"

"Cared." Jeremy answered. This time "scared" came out like "cared." Though high-pitched and not very intelligible, it was more understandable, barely.

Giving up, Heather ended the drill by using our standard-ending phrase with an upbeat, cheerful voice, "Go play." As Jeremy left, Heather turned to Crystal with a raised eyebrow.

Crystal answered her wordless question. "Come back to that emotion when he can articulate the word *scared* better, okay?" She glanced over at me. "Add 'scared' to his *Verbal Imitation* drill list." Turning from me to Randall, she requested, "Now Randall, would you like to do *Verbal Imitation*? You need to work on a list of words during *Verbal Imitation*. Add to the list random words and also words Jeremy is mispronouncing, just like we did with the word *scared*. Also, you need to practice random phrases. I think he is up to three syllables."

"Okay." Randall called Jeremy back to the room. He rotated in his chair and started *Verbal Imitation*. "Go Cowboys."

Jeremy attempted the phrase, and Randall rewarded him.

"Beat Packers," Randall urged with a mischievous glimmer in his eyes.

Zach chuckled, and Heather and I looked at each other and giggled. Always businesslike, Crystal, who was from Wisconsin, the land of the Green Bay Packers, ignored it. Randall wanted to get a rise out of Crystal but didn't succeed. Maybe Crystal was ignoring bad behavior.

I smiled. Randall's sense of humor had come back, and so had mine. For the moment, the solemn atmosphere of our home had changed to one of hope and purpose. The hopelessness and chaos of life had been driven out by what I felt God had in mind all along. God had taught me to look for what was successful. With that small seed we had come to this point in our quest to help Jeremy. Having pushed past the initial heartache of Jeremy's diagnosis, we were going on with life. Though we had a great deal of work ahead, we had a definite plan to help Jeremy, and it felt good.

Randall added a few more phrases for Jeremy to repeat and dismissed him from the table.

I elbowed Heather. "We'll have to teach him to say, 'The rain in Spain falls mainly on the plain,' right?" I grinned at her, and she smiled back.

Crystal spoke to me. "Karen, you can do the 'I see' drill."

"Okay." I liked this drill. It was the first step to teach Jeremy to talk in sentences. For Jeremy we needed to break down learning into small manageable units, and this drill was a beginning. We planned to teach short easy sentences that started with "I have," "I want," and "I see."

I placed a plastic bug and a toy car on the table. "What do you see?" We had already taught this question, so I didn't give him a verbal prompt, but gave him a slight prompt by pointing to the first items I wanted him to say.

"Buh an ca," Jeremy answered.

I knew he was trying to say "bug and car," but I wanted him to say "I see a bug and a car." I looked to Crystal for guidance, but didn't wait for her to help. "Almost."

"Say, 'I see a bug and a car'."

Crystal interrupted, "You need to ask the question over. The question and the prompt should always be paired."

"Oh, right." I nodded to her and turned to Jeremy. "What do you see? Say, 'I see a bug and a car'."

"I see a bug and a car," Jeremy responded in a slightly clearer voice.

"Great talking," I gushed.

I worked on "I see" a few more times, dismissed Jeremy from the table, and then cleared off the items to get ready for the next drill.

"Zach, you start the new drill, *Conversation*." Crystal began writing down the first few items to teach Jeremy for the *Conversation* drill.

I leaned forward and watched as she wrote,
*"What is your name? Response: Jeremy."*
*"How old are you? Response: I'm three."*
*"Who's your sister? Response: Jennifer."*
*"Hi, Jeremy. Response: Hi, _____."*
*"Bye, Jeremy. Response: Bye, _____."*
*"Who loves you? Response: Mommy and Daddy."*

My attention was drawn away from her scribbling as she continued talking. "The first on the list is 'What's your name?' I understand someone taught Jeremy to respond to that question the week before the workshop. So you teach the next question, 'How old are you?' You will need to prompt him with the correct answer the first few times—then you can fade out the prompt."

The idea of Jeremy learning to have a conversation was exhilarating. It was a beginning, and all I could expect right now.

After Jeremy sat in the chair, Zach jumped right into the drill. "How old are you? Say, 'I'm three'."

"I'm three." Jeremy worked so hard to get out the two syllables it made me want to cry. His articulation of the words fell short, but he was trying so hard.

"Super."

Zach repeated the question with the prompt. When he asked the fourth time, he did not prompt.

Jeremy answered the question without the prompt. "I'm three."

Hope and apprehension warred inside me. Many of the critics of ABA therapy ask, "How can a child learn if he is only learning by rote?" I had defended the therapy in the past by saying, "It's okay to tell a child the answer if that will help him to learn." I didn't feel there was anything wrong with giving him the answer. How could it hurt?

Jeremy had been so good at generalizing what he had learned so far. Many children in ABA therapy have to work longer and harder on each item learned. The therapists make up scenarios to help the child generalize. But, watching Jeremy, I wasn't so sure learning by rote would do him any good. Did he understand the question at all?

Also, if it was so hard to articulate "I'm three," could he ever learn how to talk as well as other children? There in the middle of the long awaited workshop, for the first time in a few months I questioned whether the therapy was going to be enough. Then I reminded myself that we were doing our best— that was all we could do. The emotional war inside me subsided as hope won out. This was good.

After Jeremy left the table, Zach expressed a concern similar to mine, "Does he know what this means?"

"We will teach the meaning later. For now, he just needs to know the answer," Crystal reassured him.

"Remember, we have to break learning down in small manageable units. We will be putting it all together later, right, Crystal?" I spoke up from the sofa.

Crystal nodded. "The Same/Different drill is next. Go ahead, Karen."

"Right." I placed a block and a cup on the table.

As I walked Jeremy to the table, he threw a tantrum. Many times I had given in to his tantrums because I feared I had worked him too hard. However, knowing that giving in only caused problems in the long run, I endeavored to continue working. If I felt he needed a break, I must learn to wait until he doesn't connect quitting with the tantrum. "Quiet, Jeremy."

Though I had him in the chair, he twisted his head and body around, trying to get out of the chair. Wanting perfection before I started, I held him in the chair and urged, "Stop, Jeremy. Sit still."

Crystal leaned forward. "As soon as you say, 'quiet,' you jump right into the drill."

"Oh, I thought I had to have everything perfect."

Crystal shook her head.

"Okay." I turned back to Jeremy, picked up his hands, laid them on the table. "Hands quiet." This time instead of waiting for several seconds to have his complete concentration, I immediately gave the command while holding up a cup that matched the cup on the table. "Give me same." For a prompt, I pointed to the cup. The prompt would be faded when he had the concept.

Jeremy picked up the matching cup.

Jumping immediately into the drill worked, I got a sudden insight into one of the reasons I was having trouble keeping discipline during therapy. I was waiting for perfect attention before working, and I gave in to his tantrums. That was not the way it worked. I only needed to get his attention for a moment— then use that split second to teach him what he needed to know. I could dismiss him from the table for short breaks between drills.

The pieces of the therapy were coming together for me. The whole process worked to pull him back into the world with the rest of us. Each time we called him to the table it was like he was beckoned back from the world inside his own mind that had shut out everyone else. Making him think in appropriate ways and learn appropriate skills was like rewiring his brain.

After the three-day workshop, I began to feel more equipped for our task. I couldn't wait to start teaching Jeremy and training our other therapists in the new skills we had learned over the weekend.

# CHAPTER TWELVE:

# MISTAKES, SHARKS, AND

# ZONING OUT

A fter the first workshop, everyone who worked with Jeremy
seemed to receive a burst of energy, especially Jeremy and
me. He needed an enjoyable yet orderly atmosphere for learning.
I needed the structure as much as he did so I could keep a
consistent schedule. I felt if I could set a plan in motion, we
could make this work. Despite my tendency to procrastinate, I
couldn't let therapy fizzle out.

Jessica, a pre-med student we had hired, arrived for her
first work session the week after the workshop. She had
impressed me with her commitment to everything in her life—
her husband and baby, her college courses, and now Jeremy.
Jessica had a big heart and gave generously to Jeremy, and that
day we had a great work session with Jeremy. Like a computer
sharing information with another system, I loaded Jessica with all
I had learned during the workshop.

Crystal had showed me an easy way to document Jeremy's
progress. We had a three-ring binder with a divider for each drill.
I taught everyone the progression for introducing new items,
mixing them with mastered items, and then writing down the
results so that the next person would know what to do.

In addition to the three two-hour sessions six days a
week, I had regularly scheduled meetings with the therapists in

which we worked together coordinating drills and solving problems. I also held phone meetings with Crystal as needed.

One day not long after the first workshop, Megan, an animated, cheerful college student, came for a therapy session. About an hour into her two-hour time slot, Megan and Jeremy came walking down the hall. It was too late for the break and too early for the session to be finished. Looking down at Jeremy, I knew something wasn't right. Jeremy made slight jerking movements which was a sure sign of overload.

I gave Megan a questioning look.

Before I could ask what was wrong, Megan answered my silent question. "I worked Jeremy for a solid hour without a break, and I think it's too much." She looked down at Jeremy with a sad, sweet smile.

Anger welled up inside me. I had told her the pace to set with Jeremy. Had she not understood? Trying not to show my anger, I quickly reined in my emotions. I didn't think it would do any good to get angry. She just needed to be told more clearly. I would not have allowed her to work without supervision if I had known she didn't understand.

Attempting to keep my voice even, I said, "Megan, remember what I said? You are supposed to give him small breaks between each drill and then a fifteen-minute break after 45 minutes. He overloads if you're not careful."

"I'm sorry. I guess I can't finish my session, huh?"

"Yeah, he can't work anymore for a while. Go ahead and sign out. I'll see you next time."

Megan looked at me. "He worked so well at first, too." She walked into the dining room to sign out. As she left, she said bye to Jeremy.

After the door shut, I sighed. "Jeremy." Kneeling, I gave him a big hug. My heart ached for him. These were not the mistakes to make with him. I had to work harder to keep the therapists well-trained and up on what to do and what not to do.

I walked into Jeremy's room. Toys and therapy props were scattered all over the floor. I reached down and picked up a

A LIFE TO RESCUE

Superman action-figure and some picture cards. I needed to ask the therapists to leave the room as orderly as they found it. Sometimes I forgot to check the room before the next session. It needed to be straightened for the next person. Maybe at the next meeting, I could ask them to straighten the room at the end of their time.

Jeremy walked in and handed me a drawing of a shark.

I smiled. Jeremy loved sharks, and some of the therapists drew him animals during their time with him. "Who drew this shark, Jeremy?"

"Zach." Then Jeremy picked up some paper and a pencil. "Draw more?"

I smiled. "Good asking, Jeremy. Okay." I sat down and spent the next few minutes drawing sharks.

The phone rang, so I ran to the kitchen to pick it up. "Hello."

It was the therapist for the afternoon time slot. "Hi. This is Darlene. Um, I'm sorry. I don't think I can make my session today."

"What's wrong, Darlene? Are you okay?"

"I'm just so tired. My boyfriend and I stayed out till three this morning. Can't you do my slot?"

Her question upset me. If I could do it all, I wouldn't have hired her. "Darlene, you have the three to five o'clock timeslot. I don't schedule myself at that time of day because I spend time with Jennifer and cook supper during that time." I wanted to work with Darlene because when she showed up, she did a good job. How could I get across to her how important this was?

I heard a heavy sigh on the other end of the phone line. "Okay, I'll be there."

"Thanks, Darlene. See you then."

I hung up the phone. Some of Jeremy's therapists understood the importance of what we were doing more than others. Was there anything else that I could do to help them understand? They had all received the same training.

After a few days and a couple of mix-ups like the one with Megan, I began writing notes on yellow Post-its and placing them on each drill that needed more explaining. Many days I used the first few minutes of each two-hour timeslot to inform the therapists of issues to watch for.

For instance, when I worked with Jeremy on the *Verbal Imitation* drill, sometimes he thought I wanted him to work on conversation. He would respond instead of repeating what I said, so I named the drill "practice talking." We began *Verbal Imitation* by saying, "Jeremy, let's practice talking." He then knew to repeat our words and not respond in conversation. I didn't want to discourage him. I also wrote at the top of the *Verbal Imitation* sheet, "Never say 'no' in this drill unless he doesn't respond at all. Say: 'Pretty good' or 'try again' or a similar phrase." I believed an informative "no" was appropriate most of the time, but not for Jeremy during *Verbal Imitation*.

One day I walked down the hall and heard Heather working with Jeremy on the pronouns "I" and "you." I heard Jeremy say, "You have the block." Then Heather said, "Good. That's right, I have the block."

A sudden insight hit me. Many autistic kids get their pronouns confused. I remembered a story about an autistic boy saying, "You want a cookie" when he meant, "I want a cookie." Many autistic individuals don't understand the difference between "I" and "you". Maybe it is because they don't have a true social awareness of people. They don't understand the concept of friendship. I wondered if anyone would ever figure out the mystery.

When Heather reinforced Jeremy's correct response, "*you* have the block" with "yes, that's right, *I* have the block", it probably confused him. We were having trouble teaching Jeremy pronouns, and now I understood why. Until he had it all straight in his brain, we needed to reinforce that response by saying, "Yes, good saying, '*You* have the block.'" We flip from "you" to "I" without thinking about it, but for Jeremy, we had to be careful, or he would be confused.

While teaching verbs, we had a special challenge. I had to make sure all the therapists demonstrated the timing of action verbs according to the verb tense we were working on. Jeremy seemed to be catching on quickly and absorbing the information at a faster rate than at the beginning.

About three months after the first workshop and after 450 hours of one-on-one with Jeremy, we had all adjusted to the unusual routine. Jeremy and Jennifer took in stride people coming in and out of our home at different times throughout the day. Through our phone consultations, Crystal had added new drills, and I was excited about Jeremy's progress. His play skills had improved as he followed a therapist to eight different play stations. Skills he learned in therapy showed up spontaneously outside of therapy sessions a few weeks after he learned them, like a delayed reaction.

On some days a therapist would come in excited about something Jeremy had learned. On one such day, Jeremy and Megan walked into the dining room after therapy. "Karen?"

"Yes?" I answered from the kitchen, walking toward her, drying my hands on a towel.

"Jeremy did real well today." She opened the therapy book, smiling. "Look, he identified 'big,' 'little,' 'wet,' 'dry,' 'hot,' 'cold,' 'clean,' and 'dirty' for me from the attribute cards today. And he's only worked on this one other time." Megan, like Jeremy's other therapists, loved Jeremy and was as happy as I was when he made progress.

Smiling at Jeremy, I bubbled, "Good, Jeremy, I'm proud of you."

My emotions soared like a rocket. I read over Megan's shoulder and saw she had documented Jeremy's answers. I couldn't wait for my work session with him.

However, when it was time for my session with Jeremy, all he did was zone out. I'm sure the phrase "zone out" is not in the books on autism, but the therapists and I began using the term to describe how Jeremy acted most of the time. He would get all glassy-eyed, stare into space, and appear to be deaf.

Following my soaring feelings, facing his spaced-out behavior depressed me. My emotions plummeted. I hated this low mood. Jeremy still had a long way to go. I began avoiding the emotional highs because afterward I would get so low—I felt hopeless.

Crystal had told us to make a list of "wake up" techniques and ways to reinforce his learning, but it didn't sink in at the time. Eventually, I would come up with lists that helped get Jeremy's attention and keep things interesting.

During the rest of my work session with Jeremy that day, I set up Superman, the Buddy doll, and some stuffed animals for *Mock Preschool*. I read a story, and we made shapes with the play dough. Pretending the dolls were working with us made Jeremy smile. He enjoyed the story and playtime, but his "zoning out" had ruined my mood during the first half of the session.

I needed to control my expectations. Yes, he had made progress, but no, he hadn't arrived yet. I should be glad for all the steps he had made in the right direction, but I couldn't allow myself to get euphoric.

In the evening, Randall and I sometimes prayed and read a Bible story for the kids. Bowing my head one evening, I started into my quickie prayer mode. I call it the Bless-Mommy-and-Daddy prayers or fill-in-the-blank prayers. "Bless . . ." I sure hoped God was listening and blessing someone because as I ended the prayer, I heard myself say, "Bye, Bye, Lord." I laughed until my side ached. Boy, I was tired.

Randall, Jennifer, and Jeremy looked at me as if I'd finally lost my mind. Then Randall started to laugh. Shaking his head, he walked over to me and gave me a hug.

"Get some sleep, honey. You need some rest."

Gratefully, I crashed into bed but not before setting my alarm for 6:30 a.m. I had too much to do tomorrow. We needed another workshop, and I wanted to start preparing.

In the morning, I wrote notes to the therapists who would be working that day. I turned to the behavior section of the therapy book where, every day, each person wrote a short note about Jeremy's behavior. I began reading through the entries in the book, flipping a page every few minutes. A few of the entries stood out from the others:

**Jan. 15** – Spurts of great attention followed by attempts to zone out. I was able to keep him with me in all activities except "what's missing." Good attitude otherwise and seemed curious. *Zach*

**Jan. 16** – Colors—he got them right, but he wanted to say "I see." Jeremy had good attention while at the table, but didn't want to come to the table by himself. During playtime he made a "T" with pretzels and said, "Jesse, Jesse, 'T.'" Overall, Jeremy did very well today. *Jessica*

**Jan. 25** – First hour—Jeremy threw three fits, but eventually got used to the fact they didn't work. He worked very well after. Cooperated well in rest of lessons. In "what do you see?" with books, the other pictures on page distracted him. Did very well in 2nd hour. Very attentive today!! Counting was GREAT! *Jill*

**Feb. 6** – Jeremy worked great today! He was extremely compliant, and he remained attentive the entire two-hour session. I did notice some stimming during the last session with hands during drills. I told him "quiet hands," and he stopped but started again on next trial. *Heather*

**March 8** – Attention was better today. Jeremy talked a lot! Sometimes his talking got in the way of drills though. On first/last drill, Jeremy was great until I asked "Which was first?" then he zoned out. *Heather*

**March 28** – Jeremy was very compliant today. He seemed to enjoy therapy. However, at times he was zoning. Jeremy talked quite a bit on his own today. I was impressed with the Book Questions program. He answered, "Who is the farmer looking for?" *Heather*

**April 6** – Jeremy was great today! He is "reading" books on his own time now—it's really cute! *Heather*

I closed the book. I needed someone to be a sounding-board for me. Maybe one of my sisters had time to talk. I picked up the phone to call Liz.

# CHAPTER THIRTEEN:
# BUILDING ON OUR OWN
# NOAH'S ARK

During my phone conversation with Liz, I told her that I was pleased with Jeremy's progress and that we were planning another workshop. "As more people step forward and share their positive experiences with this therapy, more parents will be able to help their children. It's sad when I hear about people who could afford this therapy but have never been told about it."

Liz, who is a social worker in a clinic in another state, graciously listened to my ramblings about therapy. "The clinic I work for diagnosed a boy with autism last week. I tried to share what you're doing, but no one would listen to me."

"Yeah, I know. Why doesn't anyone listen?" I cradled the phone between my chin and shoulder.

"Untreated autistic children are like a candle being snuffed out early in life without a chance to shine. Or like young people dying in a car wreck in their prime," Liz said.

"Well, I'm certainly in the battle of my life. That's for sure." I glanced at my watch. "Oh, I have to get off the phone. In a few minutes Jeremy will be getting out of a therapy session, and I have to talk to the therapist about attending the workshop this coming weekend."

"Okay, talk to you later."

Hanging up, I twisted a strand of hair and whispered softly under my breath, "I'm not sure if Jeremy will make it to complete recovery, but I do know he is being transformed before my eyes. Lord, will Jeremy be okay? Please, Lord, help us."

The door from the garage into the kitchen slammed. "Hi. Who are you talking to?" Grinning, Randall looked around, exaggerating his movements, his arms full of folders, and his camera he used for work was slung over his shoulder. "You're talking to yourself now, huh?" He raised his eyebrows as he asked the rhetorical question.

His good humor softened my mood and made me smile. But my smile faded as my mind jumped back to my worries. "Do you think Jeremy is going to be all right?" I asked.

"Karen," Randall responded gently, "you keep putting in the thermometer to test Jeremy. Give him a chance. It's only been three months."

I caught on to his analogy at once. I acted like a hypochondriac who takes his temperature too often. If I had reassurance every day, it would not be enough for me. I smiled. "Okay, I get the message. I'll make an effort to back off." I sent up a prayer instead. *Okay, Lord, could You send me encouragement soon and help me to just believe? Noah in the Bible must have had it hard. But his obedience to build the ark made him part of the miracle, just as I must be part of Jeremy's miracle. What I'm doing is minuscule compared to what Noah did.*

Going into the April workshop, I knew Jeremy had progressed. I didn't need to look at the data in the therapy book to know he had improved. Could anyone else tell?

Jeremy ran in circles in the living room during the April workshop, chattering happily in nonsensical syllables. Our therapists, Heather, Zach, Megan, Darlene, Jessica, and Jill, sat on the couch, love seat, and floor. Each person worked so few hours that it took several people to make up thirty-six hours. Jill attended my church, and I had hired her at the end of January. I had hesitated to hire someone I knew because I had to be very blunt about how we conducted therapy and didn't want to offend her. But Jill was a very special person, and I knew she would understand. Jill had shoulder-length blonde hair and an amazing mix of beauty and talent. She attended college and had a part-time job at a Montessori school. Though normally a quiet person, she taught Jeremy in an energetic way.

A married couple from the autism parent support group sat on the piano bench. A local psychologist who sympathized with our therapy approach occupied a dining-room chair right inside the living room. Randall was operating the video camera in the corner of the room, and I had taken over the brick area in front of the fireplace with my notepad of questions and therapy book. Crystal sat in a chair next to me.

In order to use our time efficiently I had asked the married couple and psychologist to hold questions until break time. I didn't want a repeat of the workshop I had attended in Austin for Kayla when a professional had used up valuable time posing questions that created doubt instead of being supportive.

Jeremy stopped his dizzy circular journey to come over to me. "Come play." He reached for my hand and gave it a tug.

When Jeremy talked and interacted, I always tried to reward him and respond.

"Good talking, Jeremy, but Mommy can't come right now." I actually needed a babysitter. *Maybe a snack would help.* I went to the kitchen and came back with a bowl of crackers for him.

*Never again. Next time I'll get a babysitter.*

Fortunately, Rita, a parent visiting Jeremy's workshop, took Jeremy into the playroom and kept him entertained during the times when we worked without him.

As in the first workshop, we systematically called Jeremy to the table and worked on each drill on his list, problem-solving as we worked. Crystal gave us insight as we went along. Having so many people around distracted Jeremy. He zoned out so much I worried Crystal would not be able to see his progress.

At break time, Rita asked if our insurance company helped with the cost of therapy.

"No, there is a list of conditions our insurance will not cover, and this is one of them," I said, sad about the reminder.

"I'm hoping to get help from social security for my daughter," Rita replied.

I opened my mouth to ask her how that worked when I noticed Darlene waiting to speak with me. I put up an index finger. "Just a minute, Rita." Turning to Darlene, I smiled. "What do you need?"

"Would it be okay if I got paid today?"

"Sure. Let me get my checkbook." I tracked down the checks and Darlene's timesheet and sat down at the dining-room table. The chatter of voices came from the therapists as they visited. Rita sat with me at the table so we could resume our discussion. When Crystal walked past with a soda, I asked, "What time does your flight leave? Do we have to be concerned about how long the final session lasts?"

She gave me the time, then reassured me, "There's plenty of time after the last session. Don't worry about it."

Randall walked by and asked me, "Did you have a chance to do the bookkeeping for the business this week?"

I nodded then signed my name to the check I was writing for Darlene. When I looked up from my task, Rita shook her head. "I don't see how you do it."

Shrugging, I smiled, ripped the check out of the checkbook, and handed it to Darlene. I turned back to Rita. "Are you getting any help from the workshop?"

Rita nodded her head. "Yes. Thank you."

I really hoped Rita would be able to start therapy for her daughter soon. At our support group, we all seemed forever stuck in teaching our kids the beginning principles most preschool children learn on their own. I really hoped Rita's daughter and Jeremy could exceed this. Some autistic children did better than others, but there always seemed to be holes in their learning, speech, and social behavior.

After we resumed the workshop, Crystal introduced the drill for Jeremy to learn how to cut with scissors. I handed the blunt-end children's scissors and paper to Crystal. Within a few minutes, Crystal had Jeremy cutting paper like a pro.

Rita, who had placed her child in a traditional special ed class, looked in amazement from her husband to me. "Do you realize how hard it is to teach this? I've worked and worked with my daughter without success. It's one of the skills they expect preschool children to have, and the public school system even tests for it."

Randall came over to me. Leaning toward my ear, he whispered, "If we had Crystal coming every week, Jeremy could learn twice as fast."

I nodded vigorously. "I agree. Crystal broke down cutting with scissors into steps, and it worked. She's an expert. She even used the command, 'Do this' when I thought we would never get any practical use out of that command."

The week after the workshop I made a "Wake Up" list for the therapists to use during therapy sessions with Jeremy.
1. Blow a whistle.
2. Pat head, then rub noses.
3. Pretend your hands are butterflies that tickle Jeremy.
4. Do Itsy-Bitsy Spider.
5. Pretend to have Superman give the command.
6. Pretend to be a T-Rex.
7. Be inventive—make up silly things.

*I should also make a list of things that might reinforce Jeremy after he gives a correct response.* I pulled out another piece of paper.
1. Verbal Praise
2. Bubbles
3. Balloons
4. Food (can be a controversial solution and some people say may lead to eating disorders)
5. Noisemaker

For other children these lists would look different, but for Jeremy this was a good start.

Retrieving the therapy book, I reached for the yellow Post-its to write a note for the animal sounds drill. I had probed with questions like "What does a cat say?" and found out Jeremy already knew eighteen animal sounds without being taught. Because he knew this concept, the drill continued by teaching the reverse of the questions, for example, "What animal goes meow?" Now he could successfully answer about fifteen animals.

We needed to find out if Jeremy had gotten the concept of this drill by asking him to answer a question he had never been taught. After any drill where Jeremy had achieved fifteen to twenty items in a program, we had to find out if he had generalized the concept taught in the program. First, we asked an untaught question in that program. If he could answer a unique question and respond to different people in different locations, then he probably had generalized the knowledge in that drill. Our consultant let us know when he was ready for different steps. All these things would broaden his ability to use what he had learned.

I flipped my pen against the table and twisted a strand of hair. Um, in the future I think I'll leave several items untaught so that after he's mastered fifteen items, I'll have some questions available to ask him. I need to make sure he has generalized the knowledge. For animal sounds, maybe I can ask him, "What animal goes oink-oink?" We haven't taught pig yet.

\*\*\*

Every few weeks, Melissa, Kayla's mother, would call me from Austin, or I would call her. Melissa spent much of our conversations questioning Crystal's abilities. I couldn't get over how opposite our experience had been with Crystal.

Melissa said things like, "I don't understand what good the building drill does. . . . I think she's too young to know what she's talking about . . . What good is the *Nonverbal Imitation* drill?"

Attempting to be diplomatic, I would just tell Melissa our experience and why I thought certain drills or concepts were important. One thing that puzzled me was her questioning simple drills as if they were somehow beneath Kayla's abilities. Kayla couldn't answer *any* questions. Why not start with the simple and build up? I really hoped Melissa would catch on soon for Kayla's sake.

Would all those professionals that attended Kayla's workshop get a true picture of what this therapy was all about? It worried me, but I would probably never know.

# CHAPTER FOURTEEN:
# CANDYLAND, ANYONE?

In May, about five months into therapy and after about seven hundred therapy hours with Jeremy, we added new drills such as *Games, Be Teacher*, and *Statement-Statement*. It felt good to have the review notebook grow larger as Jeremy mastered old drills. It gave me a sense of accomplishment.

The behavioral management techniques worked well when paired with the learning. Inappropriate behaviors like Jeremy's hand flapping began to fade as we directed him in appropriate learning. Also, Jeremy was developing relationships with the therapists. Both accomplishments were wonderful byproducts of the therapy. Although we would be working more in the future on his social skills, seeds of interacting with others had taken root in his life. In the past, Jeremy's world had shut out everyone but me. Now he had let others into his world. I'd see Jeremy talk and interact with Heather and the other therapists at break time, and I was encouraged each time.

Though working on pronouns and prepositions continued to be difficult for Jeremy, other things like the *Pretend* drill were easy for him. He loved to pretend to be an airplane, holding up his arms and zooming around the room. He also enjoyed *Complex Instructions*, which sometimes involved going into other rooms.

When we introduced the preschool game, Candyland, the first game in the *Games* drill, I thought he might never learn how to play. Jill and Jessica, two of our therapists, and I tried to teach him "pick a card," "I've got (card color)," and "move to the next square," starting with the last ten squares on the game board. It didn't work. I added to my list of questions for Crystal: how do we get Jeremy to respond to the "*Games*" drill?

One day at the end of May, I went into Jeremy's room for a therapy session—a twin-size bed with an ABC design bedspread sat at one end of the room and matching curtains hung in the windows. A preschool table and chairs had been pushed to one side. On the wall nearby, shelves held therapy props such as picture cards, etc., used for teaching Jeremy. I set the therapy book on the floor and pulled the two chairs to the open space in the middle of the room. Sitting down in a chair, I pounded playfully on the other chair. "Jeremy, come sit down."

Jeremy smiled and sat down. A sense of satisfaction coursed through me at his response. He was enjoying therapy.

I started on the newest conversation drill. "I like to eat chicken nuggets."

"I like to eat French fries," he said. Teaching Jeremy the give and take of conversation in small segments was a great building block for him. Step by step we had taught him, and he responded according to the categories we used in our sentences. I had always taken for granted the mechanics of reciprocating conversation. If someone were to ask me, "How do you teach conversation?" I couldn't have answered. But with the help of our consultant, this seemed a logical place to start. We taught him appropriate responses to simple statements people make every day.

"Good talking, Jeremy." Continuing with another item, I said, "I like to drink orange juice."

"I like to drink milk," Jeremy said, placing an elbow on the table and putting his chin in the palm of his hand.

I picked up the bubbles and blew bubbles in the air as a reward for an appropriate reply. "Good job." *What previously mastered statement could I mix in? Oh, I know.* "My favorite color is blue."

Jeremy gave me eye contact. "My favorite color is red."

I blew more bubbles and cheered, "Great talking." We worked on a few more statements. Then in an upbeat voice, I said, "Go play."

I wrote the results in the therapy book and turned the page to the *Be Teacher* drill in the notebook. "Jeremy, come here. *Be Teacher* for '*What's Missing*.'"

A happy spark illuminated Jeremy's eyes. He ran over to the table and started placing items on the table—a toy soldier, a block, a plastic bug, and a toy car—then turning to me, he commanded, "Sit down, Mommy."

"Okay." I sat down.

Giving me an all-knowing look, he took the soldier off the table and hid it behind his back. "What's missing?"

Scratching my head, I pretended to contemplate the question and then replied, "The soldier."

"Very good," he rewarded in an excited, cheery voice. Smiling, he put the soldier back and removed the block. "What's missing?"

This time I decided to miss the answer. "The car."

"No. Try again," he said in his cute little boy voice.

"Oops. I mean, block."

"Very good," he praised again, sounding joyful and happy that I had gotten the right answer.

"Can I go play now?" I asked.

"No," he answered then continued the drill until I thought I would completely wear out. Finally, he bubbled, "Go play." He walked over to the therapy book and started scribbling the "results" of the drill. I let him mark up a whole page and thanked him. We had never taught him to "write" in the book, but he had seen us write in the book after each drill so he emulated us. What a cutie and what progress!

I went on to work with him on past tense verbs, pronouns, and prepositions. He began to "zone out," but then I got his attention again during *Drawing*, *Categories*, and *Rooms-of-the-House*.

Because many autistic children lack appropriate toy play and group learning skills, we had a *Playtime* and *Circle Time* planned for each day. Both activities took about 30 minutes, so the morning therapists worked on play and the afternoon people worked on circle time. Since I had the morning session, I started playtime. For thirty minutes, we played hide & seek, big blocks, train, grocery store, and Cookie Monster. Then I went to Jennifer's room and got her Barbie and Ken dolls and handed Ken to Jeremy. Lifting Barbie, I said, "Hi, Ken."

Jeremy lifted Ken up to Barbie. "Hi, Barbie."

Improvising, I glanced around the room. Seeing a plastic snake on the floor, I got an idea. In my best damsel-in-distress voice, I breathed, "Oh, Ken, look, there's a snake. I'm scared of snakes. Help me."

"It's okay. I'll help you." Jeremy walked Ken over to the snake, picked it up, and put it in the toy box.

"Oh, thank you, Ken. You're my hero."

After playtime we walked together through the house. I put the therapy book where we kept it in the dining area, and Jeremy went into the kitchen. He looked in the pantry and then in the refrigerator. "You need to go to the store, Mommy." Giving me a stern look, he left the room.

Randall found me laughing in the kitchen. "What is it?" he asked as he looked in the refrigerator for something to eat.

"We have no food, and even Jeremy is telling me to go to the grocery store. Coming from Jeremy, that's really something. He's never communicated that well before."

"Is this a new therapy technique to get Jeremy to talk? Starve-the-family method, huh?" Randall teased, giving me a big grin.

Glancing at my watch, I saw that the kids and I had time to go to the grocery store before the next work session.

At the store I placed Jeremy in the cart's child seat and moved past the pharmacy with Jennifer trailing along beside the cart. "Oops. I forgot to get shampoo." I saw the shampoo about halfway down the aisle within visual range. "Jennifer, stay here and guard Jeremy."

"Okay." She started marching up and down next to Jeremy with her arm up holding an invisible rifle like a soldier on watch. A lady walking by laughed at Jennifer as she continued her "guard duty."

Smiling, I walked backward so that I could keep an eye on the kids and reached down and got a bottle of shampoo. When I returned to the cart, I dropped the bottle with a thump and looked up to see Linda from the autism parent support group.

"How's it going, Karen?"

"Hi," I responded with a welcoming smile. Standing next to Jeremy and Jennifer, I went on to tell Linda about therapy. Then I asked her how her autistic son was doing.

While we talked, Jennifer made silly faces at Jeremy and started to jump up and down next to the cart.

Jeremy laughed, leaned toward Jennifer, and looked at her as she continued with her silly antics.

Linda took in Jeremy's reaction to Jennifer and bragged, "Good interaction, Jeremy."

I smiled. Only moms like Linda and I thought about interaction and rewarding it. It made perfect sense to us. Though Linda hadn't witnessed Jeremy using any language she knew his eye contact and his reaction to Jennifer were social responses, behaviors that were absent in many autistic children. Yes, Jeremy had made progress.

The end of the school year arrived. Many of our therapists called in asking for time off to study for final exams. At first I worked the extra hours, but I quickly burned out. I really needed to pace myself to keep up therapy over the next few years. I had no idea how long Jeremy would need to get through all the programs available. Fortunately, I found some therapists who were willing to increase their hours during times others could not work.

Occasionally one of the therapists would question why we needed to teach a particular program. One day I asked Vicki to introduce the *Choice* program. Vicki, an attractive, high-energy woman in her forties, worked about three sessions a week with Jeremy. Most of our therapists were young adults or still in college. Vicki didn't fit that mold, but she was nevertheless committed to Jeremy.

"What is the purpose for the *Choice* drill? I don't understand what good it will do," Vicki questioned. I explained the new program to her. Since Vicki had three of her own children and none had developmental problems, she couldn't relate.

I had gone through this before, not for this exact drill, but with other therapists who questioned other programs we had introduced to Jeremy. Pausing a moment, I deliberated on the best way to explain it to her. "Did you ever see the movie *Rainman* in which Dustin Hoffman plays an autistic man?"

"Yes," she said with a slight nod of her head.

"Do you remember the scene when Tom Cruise's character wanted his autistic brother to come live with him, and the doctor asked Dustin Hoffman's character, 'Where do you want to live, in the hospital or with your brother?' Do you remember what the autistic brother does?"

Vicki shrugged her shoulders.

"He overloads, starts rocking, and then echoes the question over and over. One problem many autistic people have is they can't make a choice." I opened my mouth to continue trying to clarify when Vicki raised her hand, stopping the flow of words.

"I understand now," she said. "No need to explain anymore." She picked up the therapy book and walked over to where Jeremy was playing. "Come on, Jeremy." Then they walked into Jeremy's room to work. The set of her shoulders sent a message of renewed determination and understanding.

I believed she understood.

Breathing a sigh of relief, I turned to my notepad and reviewed the issues I needed to discuss with Crystal. I had scheduled a phone consultation with her when I knew Jeremy would be working with someone else.

After a few minutes, I connected with Crystal on the phone. "We are having trouble getting him to understand how to play Candyland. Do you have any ideas?"

"Yes, as a matter of fact, I do," Crystal said.

Pulling Jeremy through every piece of learning was important to me. Playing board games mattered—the turn-taking if nothing else. And other children played board games. He needed to learn this.

Working with Jeremy and seeing him interact meant the world to me. Each program seemed to jumpstart a piece of development that most people took for granted. Jeremy needed this.

# CHAPTER FIFTEEN:
# SOCIAL INTERACTION WITH
# KIDS JEREMY'S AGE

How many mothers in America care one way or the other whether their child can play Candyland? I'd say not many. In my case, I wanted Jeremy to learn—it was all a part of being a kid.

During my conversation with Crystal, she told me to draw a few big squares on a poster board and use that for the game board until he understood the concept. "If that doesn't work, call me, and we'll come up with a new idea."

Having a huge board with fewer squares made sense to me. It was worth a try.

Normally I didn't leave during a therapy session. If Jeremy needed something or the therapist had a question, I wanted to be there. That day, however, I asked Vicki if she cared if I left to buy something at Wal-Mart.

Vicki said it was fine, so I hurried out to purchase the poster board. When I arrived home I immediately started to work on the giant-sized Candyland game board. I drew eight huge connecting squares on the poster board and colored them different colors. The board looked good, and I had it ready for the next session.

The poster board idea worked, and we taught Jeremy how to pick cards for his turn, how to move on the board, and how to verbalize what color cards he had chosen. We were soon able to use the regular Candyland game board. At each session, a therapist would prompt him and show him how to play the game while working simultaneously on the fourteen other programs. About a month later, in June, Jeremy said to Heather, "I got the idea. Do board game." Since all the therapists had been taught to reward and reinforce any talking or interaction, Heather immediately played Candyland with him.

After Candyland, we introduced the game, Hi Ho Cheerio. He learned to play Hi Ho Cheerio in the first session and in two days he played Hi Ho Cheerio like a pro. From then on, he got the concept of any board game we introduced in the first sitting. We went on to introduce Willie Go Boom, Location Lotto, Animal Dominos, Alphabet Soup, and Potato Pals. Every time I went to the toy store I looked for a preschool game to bring home for Jeremy. Normally I wouldn't have spent so much money on games, but Jeremy's development and learning had become a top priority in our lives and finances.

In another phone consultation, Crystal informed me, "It's time to talk about peer play for Jeremy. He is ready now. Schedule thirty minutes the first time and build up to fourteen hours a week. The peer play time counts as part of your therapy time with Jeremy. I'll send instructions in the mail."

I jotted down notes while she discussed peer play with me. "Okay," I mumbled, continuing to scribble as fast as I could.

"Also, I believe he'll be ready for preschool this fall. You will have to build time slowly for him. One of the therapists will need to be a shadow. The therapist needs to reinforce him when he is doing well and prompt him when he needs to interact or attend to a task or whatever. Then they will need to fade prompting until there is no need for a shadow at all."

One day the phone rang. The woman on the line introduced herself as the parent of an autistic six-year-old boy. "I understand you are using an intense therapy approach for your son. Can you tell me about it?" she asked.

"Sure." I immediately summarized what we were doing for Jeremy—how many hours we worked, how many employees we had, and how we flew in a consultant approximately every three months from Wisconsin to supervise the therapy. "Jeremy is making so much progress." I told her Jeremy's response to doing the *Be Teacher* program. We had been so discouraged when Jeremy was two years old, barely talking or interacting, but now seeing him learn and grow, thrilled us. I wanted her to know the therapy was effective and successful for us and many others.

At the end of our discussion, to my dismay, I discovered she had no intentions of starting therapy. "We have our son in special ed. He doesn't have any extra time for therapy."

Since she had called me, I felt I should make an attempt to tell her special ed wasn't going to be enough. "How many autistic kids reach normal functioning from special ed?"

"Well, I really don't see how I can pull him out of his current class. The teacher is really nice."

I wanted to say more to this mother. However, it was her decision, not mine. "Well, if you ever want to talk about therapy more or you have questions, give me a call. I'll help you if I can."

We ended the phone call, but I wished I had said more. I didn't want to push my will on others, but at the same time, I wanted them to know the facts. How many times had I heard a parent from the autism support group tell how she had discovered her child sitting flapping her hands or engaging in some other self-stimulatory behavior in special ed class? If the child didn't bother anyone, the teacher just left the child alone. A teacher couldn't possibly put forth the effort we were making for Jeremy. Special ed teachers had other kids to worry about. I had a whole team just for Jeremy. Did the mother know that autistic children pick up behaviors from other autistic kids? Our kids needed good role models.

If I could give advice to other parents, I'd say, "I know that overcoming the grief and stress of having a child with a developmental delay is a challenge. But first put her through therapy until she has the language and skills needed to enter school." I understood some did not have the resources, but others, like my husband and me, had made it a matter of priority. The child's future was at stake, as well as that of the whole family. If not enough time is invested in rehabilitating a young child, the family could be taking care of their loved one for a lifetime.

We continued working almost 40 hours a week, Monday through Saturday. Part of that time we worked on *Mock Preschool* with Jeremy, along with many other programs. From the first workshop in January until August, we had labored hours with him on *Story Time*, *Crafts*, various language drills, and more. We would be working many more hours for months on these skills. Much preparation was required in order for Jeremy to enter school and be left on his own. Each kid was different. We had been told that some children would never make it. For me this was hard to accept. I hoped Jeremy would reach normalcy, but I knew there were no guarantees. At least my husband and I were doing everything within our power to help him. I didn't know of any better therapy options. In a few weeks he would enter preschool, and we would slowly phase in the hours he attended school so that he could handle being with other children and adults at school.

Along with keeping one-on-one therapy going, I started working on lining up kids for peer play with Jeremy. The consultant had told me other parents had commented that peer play was one of the hardest phases of therapy to implement. I couldn't imagine working up to 14 hours a week of peer play, but we would certainly try. Where would I find enough children with willing parents to work with me?

Zach, one of the therapists, had an adopted sister about a year older than Jeremy. She became Jeremy's first peer. Excited about this important step, I scheduled Zach to work and bring his sister for a peer play session. We would start for thirty minutes and build up incrementally with the time.

Day after day of therapy, Jeremy worked in his sessions. I was pleased when he worked because I knew Jeremy's time was spent doing appropriate tasks. Between therapy sessions, if I walked by and found him staring into space or playing oddly with his toys, I guided him toward a suitable activity such as building a Lego toy. It became a 24/7 job. So I redirected him into appropriate activities, therefore stopping the behavior. Unwanted behaviors had already begun to fade from Jeremy. But I didn't always have the energy to redirect and sometimes I couldn't think of anything to tell him to do. What do you tell a four year old to do?

***

Once again I was interviewing for a therapist position. We had people come and go, and because of the summer break I was short on therapists. This particular day, an older woman named Debbie (not her real name) came to inquire about the job. I went through my regular questions and received references. Then I gave her some training tapes and set up a time to work with her. "Debbie, there is a workshop scheduled soon." I discussed the date for the workshop and the importance of attending the workshop. When she left I realized I forgot to ask for a six-month commitment.

*Oops, it's too late to ask for a six-month commitment. I've already hired her. We'll see.*

In the evenings, Randall and I talked over some of Jeremy's current issues. One night after Jeremy had gone to bed I had my "to do" list and the therapy book spread out on the dining room table. "Guess what, Randall? I talked to the director at Jennifer's school, and she is going to let me start Jeremy in the fall with a shadow. She accepted my request well, but Jeremy will have to be toilet-trained. I've put off toilet-training as long as I can, but we'll have to face it soon."

"What does the consultant say about potty training?"

"You know it's one of the only things our consultant says they aren't very successful with. I think she said their approach works for potty training about 25% of the time. That's pretty honest, isn't it?" I reached for a Post-it to add a note to one of the programs for the next day's work. "I'm thinking of modifying the different methods I've read about to come up with something."

119

"Okay. If there is some way I can help, let me know."

"Thanks, honey." I stood up and gave Randall a big hug.

\*\*\*

During the training session with Debbie, I had her watch me work with Jeremy. I demonstrated the *Statement-Statement* program, where I said a statement to Jeremy like "I like chicken nuggets," and he responded back to me.

Glancing at Jeremy, I sighed. Jeremy looked cute in his blue T-shirt and shorts. Between drills he played with his plastic animals and happily chattered to himself.

I then showed Debbie some other programs. I told her how we rotated *Mock Preschool* and *Play Time* because of the time-consuming nature of the activities within those programs. Both took about 30 minutes to complete. When I turned the page for *Functions*, I showed her the progression of the items. "See, at the end of February, we taught *Functions* receptively. For example, I put on the table items like a book, block, car, telephone, and cup, and say, 'Give me something you read with' or 'Give me something you build with,' etc."

Debbie glanced at the documentation and nodded.

I continued, "He knew most of the receptive items without teaching him." I pointed to the next step on the sheet. "We taught him to respond to, 'What is a car for?', 'What is a pen for?', 'What is a book for?', 'What is a fork for?', 'What is a phone for?' etc."

I moved my finger down the page to show the rest of the list. Pointing to the next column, I said, "We taught the reverse of this, 'What do you drive in?', 'What do you write with?', 'What do you read with?', 'What do you eat with?' etc. We have also taught the group of questions such as 'What do you see with?', 'What do you smell with?', 'What do you hear with?', 'What do you taste with?' etc. Today, we need to teach, 'What do you blink with?'"

I turned to Jeremy. "Jeremy, come sit down."

Jeremy ignored me. I walked over and took his hand. "Come here."

This time Jeremy came without resistance.

Once we sat down and faced each other, I asked, "What do you blink with? Say, 'my eyes.'"

"My eyes," Jeremy responded.

"Super, that's right!" I put my hand up for high five, and he returned it, smiling.

I repeated the question and the prompt a few times until I felt he knew the answer without a prompt.

I turned to Debbie. "You try now. Do the *Functions* program and ask him the same question. When we think he knows it, we will mix this question with other questions in the same program."

Debbie sat in front of Jeremy's chair and asked, "Jeremy, what do you blink with?"

I peeked over Debbie's curly, blonde hair at Jeremy's face. He was zoning out, an aspect of Jeremy's disability that we still hoped to overcome.

To my surprise, Debbie retorted with a loud, harsh "no" right in Jeremy's face.

Immediately, I corrected her. "Debbie, I'm sorry, I forgot to tell you. That training video has an obsolete facet about it. The harsh ways of saying no in the tape are not done now." I paused, collecting my thoughts. "That is not the way the therapy is done now, and *we* certainly don't do therapy that way. From now on if he doesn't get the right answer, give him a nice, sweet, informational 'no,' okay?"

"But that's the way the video did it," she snapped back at me.

*What? What's the deal here? How do I handle this?*

# CHAPTER SIXTEEN:

# THE LIGHT AT THE END OF THE TUNNEL

I didn't like Debbie's reaction. *She thinks the experts haven't changed. She doesn't know how much time I spent with our consultant or how much I've read. Well, who cares, I decide what we're going to do.* Not only was I following instructions, but it was common sense to handle Jeremy with kindness. I had six people working with Jeremy. I didn't want any of us using harsh methods for handling him. It needed to be fun and rewarding for him to learn and work.

I scowled at Debbie and wondered what I should say to her. I knew if she kept this up I would have to fire her. Was I expecting too much? No. Doing my best to explain, I again related the way to handle Jeremy, and we ended the session.

With another workshop coming up within days, I made sure everyone knew the date and could attend. I made motel reservations for the consultant and planned and shopped for the food.

In the midst of the preparation, Vicki's husband Philip called. My first thought was that Vicki was sick and would not be able to attend the workshop. But Philip had something else in mind. "Karen, I really want Vicki to go with me this weekend to visit my brother-in-law. Can she miss the workshop?"

I shook my head in disappointment. I'd worked hard to coordinate everyone's schedule. The money, time, and effort would be wasted if my team didn't benefit from the workshop.

What did Vicki want? I thought we had an understanding. Most important of all we needed to impact Jeremy. His chance of recovery was at risk. I needed Philip to understand.

"Philip, you don't understand. We have—" I froze up, struggling to put into words the flood of reasons why the workshop was so important. "We are flying in the consultant. Vicki needs to be there. I don't think—"

Before I could explain why I needed Vicki at the workshop, Philip interrupted, "I understand. Vicki is stressed about working in front of everyone during the workshop. I want to help her."

Again the list of reasons rushed to my lips, and I opened my mouth to say: *Jeremy needs this. We have the consultant for just two days. We were spending about $1500 dollars to make this weekend happen. Please understand.*

All of a sudden I heard mumbling over the phone line then Vicki's voice. "Karen, don't worry. I'm coming to the workshop. I made a commitment to be there, and I will. Don't worry about Philip. I'll explain it to him."

I sighed in relief. "Thanks, Vicki."

As I hung up the phone, my stress eased with the realization Vicki had a vision of what we were trying to accomplish. She would be at the workshop. Thankfully, Philip and I had had no angry words. We had discussed everything calmly. But frustration still lingered in the air. I decided it didn't matter. Vicki would work this out. I couldn't possibly make everyone understand anyway.

Peer play began to fill some of Jeremy's therapy hours. I scheduled one of the therapists or myself to be on hand so we could prompt or reward him during playtime when needed.

We learned immediately that working the right amount of time was important. Jeremy's first peer play session with Hannah went a little too long and overloaded him. He acted like he did when he worked too much. He made little jerking motions.

One day after Jeremy had had about eight peer play sessions, Kelly, a friend from church, brought her son Ben for peer play. I had my list of planned activities. "Okay, boys, sit down for story time." Reaching for a story book, I read to them. They looked so cute, sitting cross-legged in front of me. Neither one of the boys had a clue that all these activities were planned. Since they both cooperated so well, I had *Circle Time* with *Statement-Statement*.

"I like vanilla ice cream," I said.

"I like vanilla ice cream, too," Jeremy responded back.

"I like chocolate," Ben said.

I kept the boys talking about the food they liked a little longer. We then played Animal Dominoes, Hide & Seek, and Follow the Leader. Jeremy started tickling Ben during Ring Around the Rosies. Then they took turns hitting the ball on the T-Ball stick.

Later I set up some toys in various places in the living room, hoping Jeremy would ask Ben to play. I wasn't disappointed. Jeremy walked up to Ben. "Do you want to play Batmobile?"

"Good asking, Jeremy!" We had worked for this. Wonderful!

On the other hand, I soon found out that peer play didn't always run as smoothly as that day with Ben.

During a phone conversation with my sister Mary, I told her about a peer play hazard I had encountered. "Jeremy asked a kid to play Potato Pals the other day, and the child responded, 'No, I don't want to.' How can you tell a four-year-old how hard we worked to teach Jeremy to enjoy and initiate toy play? I know how impractical it is to expect a child to understand. In spite of what I know in my head, my heart can't bear the hurt. I'm going to schedule our therapists to work during peer play sessions as much as possible. I'm way too emotionally involved."

"That's a good idea."

A slight pause interrupted our conversation. I doodled on a notepad then lined up the salt and pepper with the vitamin jars.

*I should get off the phone. I have a therapy session coming up in a few minutes.*

"Guess what, Karen? I had a dream that Jeremy was talking and singing with the family. He looked a little older than the age he is now. Isn't that neat? It seemed like a dream from the Lord," she said with a smile in her voice.

My eyes filled with tears that spilled out down my cheeks. "I've been praying again for some reassurance. Thanks for telling me." I clung to the story of my sister's dream as if I'd been thrown a lifeline.

\*\*\*

The scheduled workshop finally arrived. Two of our previous therapists, Jessica and Stephanie, who had moved to Austin, asked if they could come back to work some hours with Jeremy on the weekends. Amazed, I gladly welcomed them back. What a blessing to have these young women willing to commute two hours, round trip, to work with Jeremy. They had truly come to love him.

As we waited for the consultant to start the workshop, each one of the therapists had found places on the couch, love seat, chair, and floor. Stephanie sat on the floor near me.

Juggling papers in my lap, I asked, "Stephanie, are you getting used to Austin traffic yet? How did your move go?"

"Everything is going fine, thanks. Oh, and thank you for hooking me up with Melissa. She hired me to work with her autistic daughter."

"Where are you working?" Heather asked.

"Melissa is the parent doing the same kind of therapy for her daughter as Karen is for Jeremy. Karen introduced me to them, and I've started working a few hours a week. Jessica is working for them too."

I looked at Heather. "Melissa has the child I was telling you about who threw tantrums during most of her workshop when Randall and I visited."

Heather nodded. "Oh, yeah, I remember now."

I turned back to Stephanie. "I'm glad things are going well." I stuck my pen in the flap of the notebook, the room momentarily silent. "Does anyone want a cola or snack before we start? Please, help yourself anytime."

"Yes, thanks." Stephanie jumped up and went into the kitchen.

I leaned toward Heather on the love seat. "How did your wedding go yesterday?" I knew Heather had attended a friend's wedding and made the trip back for the workshop.

Debbie, our newest therapist, who had only been with us a few days, looked at Heather in shock. "Did you get married yesterday?"

A round of giggles rippled around the room. "No," Heather spoke up.

"Yeah, I made her come on her honeymoon," I joked.

Another current of laughter waved over the room.

Heather smiled. "It was for an old roommate's sister."

"I did word that badly, didn't I? Sorry," I apologized, laughing.

The consultant nodded at me to indicate she was ready to begin, so I spoke up, "Attention, everyone." The rumble of voices grew silent. "I think I told y'all that Crystal, our previous consultant, had the opportunity to go into research. This is Kristie Ramseier, our new consultant."

Kristie smiled at everyone.

"She has been trained at UCLA, and I'm looking forward to all the help she is going to give us." Then I introduced everyone around the circle. "Before we start, I'd like to pray."

I hoped everyone felt comfortable with prayer, because Randall and I had decided we needed prayer before workshops. We wanted God's blessing. We couldn't do this without Him.

Everyone seemed to accept my praying. After the prayer, we started.

"Before we go through some drills with Jeremy, how are things going in general?" Kristie asked.

"He improved in just the week I was gone on vacation," Heather said.

The speed at which Jeremy had progressed encouraged me and gave me hope. Jeremy's speech needed work, and many other concepts had to be taught, but he was learning quickly.

"How are his tantrums?" Kristie questioned.

"Tantrums no longer bring things to a grinding halt. But he still has one every so often," I answered, picking the therapy book off the floor in case I needed it.

"Remember, if you have trouble with tantrums, it's probably because someone is giving in to his tantrums."

I nodded my head. "I remember something good that happened the other day. Jeremy and I were building with Legos, and I said, 'I'm making a table.' He responded back, 'I'm making a car.' Doesn't that mean he's learning to apply what he's learned in therapy to out of therapy, regular situations?" I gave Kristie a hopeful smile.

Kristie smiled back. "Yes, that's good."

"We are having trouble with some of the conversation drills because he can only say about seven syllables and then he can't go on," I said.

"Go back down to six syllables until he's ready."

"Okay."

We began taking turns working on drills with Jeremy, Kristie making suggestions and correcting us when needed. Jeremy would leave between drills to play in the other room.

When Debbie's turn arrived, she placed a book and a plastic bug on the table. "Give me bug first and book last."

Jeremy gave her the bug first and then the book.

Everyone clapped. "Good job, Jeremy. What did you give me first?"

"Book."

"No," Debbie belted out harshly.

Jeremy flinched.

My heart sank. *Oh, no, I thought I handled this already.*

I opened my mouth to correct her when Kristie spoke up, "Debbie, we don't correct a child in that manner, especially one who is working for you as hard as he is."

*All right!* Kristie's tone and attitude were perfect, with just the right firmness and politeness, and though Debbie tried to make excuses, she accepted the correction. I'm glad Debbie hadn't worked for us long. It hurt to think Jeremy had had some sessions with Debbie when she treated him this way.

I would have to fire Debbie if she didn't listen this time. She had been told twice plainly. If she didn't comprehend now, she never would.

Debbie finished the drill, and Jeremy left to play in the other room.

When the time came for the *Occupation* drill, I dug out the pictures of various types of people—farmer, fireman, doctor, teacher, etc. I had purchased a box of pictures at the educational supply store that showed pictures of people dressed like many of the main professions. Later I found a poster of professions at the educational store that worked even better. I cut out each picture so we could present to Jeremy one at a time.

"The doctor and fireman are women in the pictures," I said. "I wish they had gone ahead and had men in the photos. I want him to learn that traditionally men have been in these positions. Of course," I laughed, "right now he has a female pediatrician."

"Hey, see, there you go," one of the young women said. "It's okay for women to be in the pictures."

I shrugged and laughed to let everyone know not to take me too seriously. "Okay, you're right."

Everyone laughed. Sometimes Zach, the only guy in the group, got into good-natured arguments with the girls. They'd write notes to each other in the therapy book. But this time Zach seemed to be on the girls' side.

Stephanie worked on the *Conversation* drill with Jeremy. "I have red hair."

Jeremy touched his head. "I have dark blond hair."

She continued the drill.

When they finished and Jeremy left the room, Kristie asked, "What's this with the dark blond hair?"

I laughed. "Well, we couldn't agree on what color his hair was, so I came up with that answer."

Kristie smiled. "Right, maybe you should teach him, 'I have dirty-blond hair.'" Laughter sounded in the room.

Stephanie and Zach, who both had red hair, had a discussion about different shades of red hair. They wondered if it confused Jeremy that they both claimed to have red hair when in reality one had orange hair and the other almost strawberry-blond.

We worked on more drills. Soon the discussion turned to other children who had received ABA therapy and had made it to normalcy. Megan asked, "Is Jeremy going to be one of the kids that makes it?"

We all looked at Kristie, and everyone in the room seemed to hold their breath.

# CHAPTER SEVENTEEN:
# EXPANDING CONVERSATION
# AND THE SCHOOL SEARCH

All we needed was a drum roll as we awaited Kristie's answer to Megan's question, "Is Jeremy going to make it?"

"It's too early to tell," Kristie said.

Everyone in the room seemed to exhale in unison.

Megan nodded acknowledgment of the information.

As for me, I refused to speculate. I knew his language and social skills were still behind other kids his age. I was weary of having him tested and taking him to doctors just to find out what I already knew. As long as our consultant had programs and we had money, we would keep working.

After the August workshop I started thinking about school. This meant I had to deal with toilet-training Jeremy. He had been mature enough for toilet-training for several months, but I hadn't wanted to face it. I was afraid he would resist. I hoped in the few days before he started school I could get everything ready. It eased my stress to know I had an understanding with the preschool director to have a shadow for Jeremy.

I drove to school for my fifteen-minute appointment with Jeremy's teacher, Ms. Carter. Each preschool parent had been assigned a timeslot, and I planned to take full advantage of my time. I had arranged for Jeremy to work at home with a therapist, and for Randall to work from his home office in case he was needed.

From the first minute I walked into the school, confusion reigned. People walked in and out of Ms. Carter's classroom while she had meetings with parents. I waited outside the door. A lady in a red shirt said to Ms. Carter, "I need to visit the school office. I'll be back in a few minutes." The lady appeared oblivious to the fact that if she left she would mess up the parent-teacher conferences that were scheduled back-to-back.

Looking expectantly to Ms. Carter, I waited for her to explain how it all worked. But Ms. Carter didn't say a word. She only frowned at the lady's back, appearing more stressed by the minute.

I walked over to the schedule posted on the wall in the hallway. *Oh, well, at least I'll have her attention during my timeslot.*

When my time arrived, I hovered near the door. Noticing me, Ms. Carter said, "I'm sorry. I'll be with you in just a minute." She turned back to another parent and continued her conversation.

"Sure, no problem," I assured her, walking away from the door to give them some privacy.

She talked a short time with the woman, said her goodbyes, and then welcomed me.

I introduced myself and jumped right into my plans. "I talked to the director a few weeks ago, and she said she would allow a shadow for Jeremy during class." I went on to explain a little of Jeremy's history, and what a shadow was. "Of course, the shadow would be a help to you and encourage the other children just like she will Jeremy. That way having a shadow in the room will seem more natural to the other children." The more I talked, the more Ms. Carter scowled. What was wrong? The director had assured me Jeremy could come with a shadow. Clearly, Ms. Carter had not been told.

A movement at the door caught my attention. I looked over to see the lady in the red shirt, smiling in the doorway. "I'm ready to talk, Ms. Carter."

What was she thinking? I searched the teacher's face, trying to read her body language. As far as I could tell, she was more ignorant than rude. Again I looked expectantly at Ms. Carter to see if she would explain to Ms. Red Shirt the way the schedule worked. To my chagrin, she mumbled to her, "I'll be with you in a minute."

Ms. Red Shirt's smile faded, but she backed out of the room.

*Good, we can finish our meeting.* I glanced at my watch—I had plenty of time. Expecting Ms. Carter to give me her full attention, I was disappointed when she kept glancing out the door nervously, fidgeting with the things on her desk.

"I'm sorry. Where were we?" she asked, her gaze shifting between me and the door. "Oh, yes, the shadow idea." Her fidgeting grew worse. "I don't like having someone watching me in the classroom when I work." Ms. Carter's manner grew more agitated as we talked about the shadow. Finally, she grudgingly agreed to have a shadow in the room. What else could she do since the director had already given her approval?

I left upset, knowing I'd have to find another school for Jeremy. No way would I allow Jeremy in an atmosphere where the teacher was unhappy with a shadow. When the time came for kindergarten, I could bring him back to this school if I wanted. In the meantime, I would look somewhere else.

Overwhelmed, I started searching for a preschool that would work with me. All the preschool teachers acted about the same. Smiling and polite at first, as soon I mentioned a shadow they gave me a resounding "no". One place said they would let Jeremy come but no shadow. Another place said they didn't have time to deal with him. Thinking I wasn't making myself plain, I would tell them again that I would pay for the shadow, plus the regular preschool fee for Jeremy to attend. I also tried to explain that the shadow was trained and would be a help to the classroom.

One day after one more rejection, heartbroken I sought out Randall. "I can't find a school for Jeremy. I might as well be looking for the right school for Jeremy from a list of every preschool in America. I feel overwhelmed, and I'm running out of options. I can't handle another refusal." Tears ran down my face.

"I'll try, Karen," he offered. Randall was as concerned as I was for Jeremy, and I was grateful for his help.

"Okay, thanks." Unwilling to get my hopes up too high, I didn't talk anymore about it, hoping and praying he'd have success.

In the intervening time, therapy and peer play sessions continued day after day.

Debbie called one day and said, "I'm too upset to come to work. On my way home from the store today I sat behind a wreck on the interstate for an hour."

"Oh, I'm sorry." Sympathetic, I opened my mouth to tell her not to worry about coming, but I sensed something else going on in her mood. *I don't think she really wants this job. I need to collect more information here.* "How long ago was this wreck?"

"It was early this morning," she said. Then she went on to explain that the traffic was awful. She didn't know or see the victims or find out if it was a serious wreck or anything other than waiting in traffic.

"Debbie, that was hours ago." I sighed. Somehow her excuse regarding the accident affecting her didn't ring true for me, and the incidents when she had been too harsh with Jeremy came to the forefront of my mind. Her voice—her attitude seemed to spell that she didn't care about the job with Jeremy. I made a quick decision. I said as calmly and politely as I could, "Look, your employment with me is not going well. You don't need to come to work anymore. I'm getting someone to replace you. I'll send you a check for what I owe you."

She didn't seem the least bit sorry when I told her, and I wondered if she was relieved that I let her go. Why did she bother to take the job in the first place? And why didn't she just quit if she wasn't interested?

***

The therapists and I began to expand the *Conversation* drill for Jeremy. One day I asked Vicki to teach Jeremy to ask questions during conversation. Halfway through the session she came to get me. "I've prompted Jeremy to ask a question, but he just answers the question."

"Huh, let's see. How can we handle this?" I picked up the therapy book. "Let's try modeling it for him. I've heard some kids don't respond to this, but I think Jeremy will." I set the book down, wrote down what I wanted Vicki to introduce, and handed it to her.

"Watch us, Jeremy." I sat down in the chair in front of Vicki, nodding for her to start.

"I like Superman," she chimed.

"I like Batman," I stated. "Do you like Batman?"

"Yes, I like Batman. He's cool," Vicki said.

Turning to Jeremy, I smiled. "Your turn."

I could tell by the sparkle in Jeremy's eyes he understood what we wanted him to do.

Jeremy sat in the chair in front of Vicki, and Vicki bubbled, "I like Superman."

"I like Spiderman. Do you like Spiderman?" Jeremy chattered back.

"Good asking. Yes, I like Spiderman," Vicki gushed.

I left them to work and walked down the hall feeling elated. Jeremy caught on to that really quickly. We had much more work that needed to be done for this drill, but we were over the biggest hurdle.

I heard the back door slam.

"Karen!" I heard Randall call out.

"What?"

"I have great news," Randall said. "I found a school for Jeremy." He set down a stack of papers in his hand. "The director has a son who has special needs and doesn't fit in at school, so she's sympathetic to our situation. She likes the idea of Jeremy being taught to go to school by having a shadow help him and decreasing the need for assistance slowly. One day Jeremy should be able to go to school by himself. I talked to the teacher also, and she seemed willing to work with us. I asked if you could visit on Thursday."

"That's fantastic! I'm so excited. It sounds perfect."

When I visited Ms. Brenda's classroom, I discovered it was ideal for Jeremy. She rewarded the kids in her class verbally just as we did Jeremy. I talked to her about the shadow, and she said, "I'm used to having an aide. I taught public school special ed before I came to teach at this preschool. I'll be glad for the help." She smiled at me.

I asked her if she would allow us to start Jeremy with 45 minutes the first time and then build incrementally until he was able to stay for the full three-hour timeslot. "No, I think it will be too distracting."

"Okay, I understand." Though one of my requests had been rejected, I left feeling much better than I had in a few days. Jeremy had a place to go to school. I signed him up for the Tuesday/Thursday class 9 a.m. to 12 noon, and our therapist Heather promised to be his shadow. Grateful, I thanked God for this answer to prayer.

Jeremy couldn't be in diapers and go to preschool. I looked at the calendar and told Randall, "I think I'm going to schedule toilet-training here." I pointed to the calendar. "Almost all the therapists are off these two days. It's not going to be easy, but I think it's for the best." Since starting therapy I couldn't remember a day except Sunday when someone wasn't coming in and out of our house. "Jeremy and I will have to practically live in the bathroom. I'm going to buy some new toys and treats for him."

"And I can set up the TV in the bathtub for him. That will make it more fun," Randall offered.

I smiled. "You can do that? That will be great. I want it to be reinforcing. Thanks for going through the trouble."

The big day came. I put stickers and toys in a drawer in the bathroom. I dried the bathtub of leftover water droplets, and Randall set up a box in the bathtub and put the television on it. I prepared to spend most of the day in the bathroom. It would be the first party I'd ever attended in a bathroom. Unsure if he would understand, I decided to explain to Jeremy about no more diapers.

I knelt down in front of him and made sure I had his attention. I explained everything in plain, simple language. He seemed to understand. Then I dressed him in big boy underwear with Spiderman pictures on them.

He had such a good time that by the end of the day the front of his shirt was covered with stickers.

When it was almost time for bedtime, he said, "Diaper?"

Interpreting that to mean he wanted to put on a diaper, I said, "No, remember you don't need a diaper anymore. You are going to use the toilet." I knew his receptive understanding was better than his verbal skills, so I hoped he grasped the meaning of what I was saying.

He fell on the floor and cried. When he saw I wasn't going to give him a diaper, he went to the toilet. I rewarded him with another sticker, then I handed him a new toy car. "Good job."

I knew the hardest part was over. All that worrying—and it ended up easier than I thought.

# Chapter Eighteen:
# Add PreSchool Two Days a
# Week to the Mix

---

In the next few days after toilet-training, we moved activities farther and farther from the bathroom. When Heather came about three days later, she had Jeremy's therapy session in the hallway near the bathroom door.

Toward the end of the session I wanted to discuss Jeremy's preschool with Heather. Walking from the kitchen to the hall, I saw Jeremy sitting in the doorway of the bathroom. Heather sat on the floor in front of him with the therapy book beside her. "Heather, when y'all are finished with therapy, can we talk about Jeremy's school schedule?"

"Sure, we are almost finished."

"Okay, thanks." I stood, leaning against the wall and watched.

Heather tickled Jeremy. He giggled. She smiled and said in an upbeat voice, "I went to McDonald's last night."

He should know this drill. I hoped he could go on with the conversation.

Jeremy grinned back and asked, "What did you eat?"

"I had a hamburger and fries," Heather answered.

Heather worked on conversation more, and then gave Jeremy a high five.

Jeremy ran down the hall to his room, and Heather and I walked to the dining room to discuss school.

"Heather, here's a sheet I made for you to take notes on." I handed her the sheet. Over to one side I had the following:

*Things to take note of at school:*

- *Attention/Eye Contact*
- *Sitting properly when the teacher asks*
- *Attitude (i.e. cooperative, focused, spacey, uncooperative)*
- *Social interactions*
- *Following directions (i.e. obeyed when called, obeyed most of the time, obeyed with prompting, seemed distracted, ignored requests)*
- *Inappropriate behaviors*
- *Activities with other children*
- *Generalizing things taught at home*
- *Transitioning between activities*
- *Greeting/farewells (for adults and children)*
- *Imitating other children*

I continued talking about the form. "The rest of the form is broken down by activity, and I've left space for you to write. See, the headings are broken up by the kids' schedule: Fellowship Room Singing, Bible Story Time & Activities, Snack Time, Bathroom Break, Craft Time, and Other."

On one particular morning, I drove Jeremy to school. We walked into the big room where all the preschool classes gathered to sing. I decided to stay and observe until Heather arrived. The children sang, and thankfully Jeremy participated. The song program we had worked on in therapy had done the job. Jeremy even did the motions. After a few songs all the children went to their separate classrooms.

Ms. Brenda, Jeremy, and the other children walked up the stairs. I followed close behind them and stood quietly a short distance from them as they sat in front of the teacher.

Ms. Brenda asked each child a question. When Jeremy's turn came, she asked, "What did you do over the weekend?"

When it looked as if he couldn't answer the question, I came up behind Jeremy, got on one knee, and spoke in his ear, "Say, 'I went to Wendy's with Papa and Grandmother.'"

Jeremy had no trouble with me prompting him and repeated, "I went to Wendy's with Papa and Granmeme."

While Ms. Brenda continued with *Circle Time* with the kids, I made a mental note to ask Kristie for a drill that would help with this kind of question.

Later on that day when I talked to Heather, she encouraged me. "Jeremy is doing so well in school that I mostly only prompt him for social interaction. He still needed prompting during playtime to enter into the activities." She pulled out the sheet for documenting his progress at school. "I had to tell him, 'quiet hands' a lot today because he had some inappropriate hand movements." She marked the date at the top of the form. "Oh, and he's the only one who can read his name on the crayon boxes." Pride in this accomplishment was evident in her voice. "When the teacher tells the children to get their supplies, he goes straight to where his name is displayed. I think he's doing really well."

"Thank you. Keep up the good work." She handed me the form, and I placed it into a notebook. "Is he singing during the song time when you're there?"

"Yes, except for once, he's been singing out and even doing the sign language the teacher taught the class."

"How is the interaction with the other children going?"

"Pretty good! He played in the sand with four other children today, and then I prompted him to ask Jasmine to ride on the seesaw. He did. He said, 'Jasmine, come here!'" Heather picked up her keys to leave. "Oh, and he played 'crash cars' with Bo."

I asked Kristie how we could improve Jeremy's ability to answer questions like, "What did you do last weekend?" She said we needed to have a more advanced version of the *Trips* drill. We already had a *Trip* program where we went to another room in the house, did an activity, and returned to his room. Then we would asked, "What did you do?"

The advanced trip program would have us take Jeremy into the community. Then when we arrived home, we asked, "What did you do?" I tried to incorporate this kind of question throughout normal activities too. If I went to the grocery store, I would use it for a therapy opportunity.

In November about eleven months and 1,500 hours into therapy, we had another workshop. Five of our therapists and Kristie, our consultant, attended. When the time came to bring Jeremy to the table to work, I started with his favorite program, hoping he would feel less self-conscious.

Sitting Jeremy in front of me, I asked, "Why do you smile?"

Smiling, Jeremy answered, "Because I'm happy." His overall speech still lacked articulation, but he had improved.

"Why do you sleep?"

"Because I'm tired," he said immediately.

"Why do you take a bath?"

"Because I'm dirty."

"That's right," I rewarded, laughing.

"Why do you hug Mommy?"

"Because I love her."

"Oh, I'm so glad." I reached for him and gave him a big hug, and the therapists let out a collective "ah" at the same time.

"Why do you go to school?"

"To eat bagels."

"Hmm, that's an interesting answer," I said, trying hard not to laugh at his creative response.

I repeated the question. "Why do you go to school? Say, 'to learn.'"

"To learn."

"Good. Why do you play with toys?"

"Because it's fun."

"That's right. Go play."

Jeremy jumped up and happily ran out of the room.

Then we discussed when Jeremy made up answers to questions other times besides his interesting answer about going to school to eat bagels.

Turning to Kristie, I explained, "When we introduced the *'I don't know'* drill, we asked him a question we knew he couldn't answer, and we were able to teach him to respond 'I don't know.' Then he asked a question to clarify what we asked about."

We decided if Jeremy gave an appropriate answer, even though it was not the answer taught, it was okay. We could reward for the answer. We did need to make sure he understood the item we were targeting for him to learn.

Heather spoke up, "The other day I asked Jeremy 'who loves you?', and he answered 'Mommy and Daddy'. He then started a whole long list of people who love him. He started naming everybody. We only taught him 'Mommy and Daddy.'"

Kristie smiled. "That's great."

The *Quantities* program came next. Jill stood up to start this program while I went back to Jeremy's room to get him and to bring some small toys to use for the drill.

When they were both ready, Jill set out on the table three piles of small plastic toys—one pile of dinosaurs, one pile of soldiers, and one pile of bugs. "Give me all the dinosaurs, some of the soldiers, and none of the bugs."

Jeremy did it.

Everyone applauded.

"Great, Jeremy!" Jill put all the toys back into three groups. "Now give me a couple of dinosaurs, none of the soldiers, and a bunch of the bugs."

Again Jeremy executed the request accurately. Jill rewarded him, and he left for his room.

"Jeremy's doing better with this program than I am. I've started having to write down what I'm doing, or I lose track," I said, laughing.

"Don't ask too many in one sitting," Kristie advised.

"I found out I need to vary the number of items I use for the words few and some. If I'm not careful he thinks few and some are the same number of items every time," Heather remarked.

We went on to discuss how Jeremy was getting "she" and "he" confused and would mix them up in conversation.

Stephanie and Jeremy worked on the *Occupation* drill.

Stephanie held up a picture of a fireman. "Who is this?"

"A fireman," Jeremy answered.

"What does a fireman do?"

"Put out fires."

"What does a policeman do?"

"Catch bad guys."

When it was my turn again to work with Jeremy, I did a program called *"What's Happening Here?"* I picked up two children's picture books. Pointing to a picture, I asked, "What's happening here?"

"They're playing in the park."

Pointing to various pictures, I asked the same question, "What's happening here?"

Each time Jeremy gave a summary sentence for each picture. "They're having a party. ... They're going to sleep. ... They're shopping. ... They're reading a book."

"Great talking, Jeremy. Go play."

At break, some of the therapists talked about their boyfriends. I needed to pray for each one of them since this was an important decision-making time in their lives. They were all unmarried except Jessica. Chris, the new male therapist, kept quiet. Zach usually talked about his girlfriend who lived in Pennsylvania.

The time came to start work again, and I stood up to get Jeremy. As I walked toward the hall, and called out, "Jeremy, come here!" I mentioned to those within earshot, "He doesn't respond when I call him from another room. That's a developmental problem I hope he overcomes."

The words had barely left my lips when I heard Jeremy call out from his room, "What?" Then he ran to me.

I made a mini-celebration out of this accomplishment. What outwardly appeared to be a small thing was huge to me. Everyone who had heard my comment started complimenting Jeremy at once and telling me I was wrong to think he couldn't do it. I smiled at everyone, and we started to work again.

Heather implemented scripted play with Jeremy. They came in the room with a couple of blankets and some string.

"Jeremy, let's go camping," Heather said cheerfully.

They acted and talked out a pretend trip to the camping ground. When they went fishing, Jeremy exclaimed, "I got a crocodile!"

A soft giggle flowed over the room. They cooked their fish and roasted marshmallows. Soon it was time to go home. Jeremy drove.

After acting out the camping trip, Jeremy left the room.

"When I led peer play the other day, Ashley insisted Jeremy drive. Isn't that cute? And they embellished other things in the story we never taught," Heather said.

"It's going well. On most of the scripted play, you need to reverse the role Jeremy acts out before you drop the game, okay?" Kristie encouraged.

The program, *Listen to a Story*, had been progressing for about two months. We had started with a little story like this: "John ran. The end." Then we asked questions like, "Who ran? What did John do?" By now we had worked up to a slightly longer story and eventually would be working up to a ten-sentence story.

Stephanie made up the story, "Jenna went to Wal-Mart and bought a doll and looked at the plants. The end." Then she asked who, what, where questions.

The programs were getting more and more complex each month, and Jeremy had completed each task we gave him. We still ran into obstacles like confusing "he" and "she" and trouble with his articulation. He also had some occasional odd behaviors like shifting his eyes in an odd way. But we were dealing with each obstacle as things arose. This was life now.

# CHAPTER NINETEEN:
# IMPROVEMENT ACCELERATES

I lived and breathed therapy so much I rarely did anything else. Life focused on Jeremy.

I adopted the philosophy, "I'll sleep when I'm dead." In other words, I'd rest or relax when therapy was all over, even if it meant waiting a few years. I said that in humor, but if you ask parents running an ABA program for their child, it isn't funny. I had met parents who had sacrificed even more than we had to run a therapy program. They sold their home or business or moved to be near a clinic just to give their child needed therapy. I heard of parents in some areas of the country paying $70,000 to $100,000 a year for therapy. Thankfully, we paid only a fourth of that amount. We were just regular middle-class Americans, far from rich. Randall worked hard to provide the money needed for Jeremy's needs. He drove an older model car he bought from my dad, and I drove an economy car. Though we spent thousands of dollars, it was worth every penny. It was like paying for a college education during preschool.

God always provided. Every time I calculated whether or not we had enough money to continue therapy, I'd come up short. Somehow we always had an adequate amount of money. Isn't God good?

One day after a therapy session, Zach walked down the hall smiling. "Jeremy talked so much today we almost didn't get all his work done. He seems to be coming out of the Christmas slump he was in."

I smiled at the idea of Jeremy talking too much. "I wonder if he was in a slump at Christmas because I never want to work at Christmas time. He probably caught my feelings somehow. I'm glad he's out of it though. Is there anything else I need to know from your session with him?"

"Yes, he doesn't want to drink out of a regular cup. He always wants a straw. The drill you made where he practices drinking out of a cup as part of therapy goes fine. But between drills he doesn't want to drink without the straw."

I didn't understand Jeremy's resistance to drinking out of a cup, so I made up a drill to encourage him to drink without a straw. One of the things our consultant had taught us was to make drills based on Jeremy's needs. I finally understood how to do that. I smiled. "Okay, I think we'll have to gradually phase in the cup without the straw. Thanks."

Zach left, and Jennifer and Jeremy ran by me on the way to the TV. Jeremy wore navy blue sweat pants and shirt—the pants pushed up to his knees and shirt sleeves pushed up to his elbows. I guess he found it more comfortable. Jennifer looked equally cute in her pink flowered shirt and matching knit pants.

"Jeremy, come watch *Magic School Bus* with me," Jennifer encouraged in a sweet voice.

I sat down at the dining table and worked through the therapy book, looking to see if Jeremy had progressed in any of his drills sufficiently to go to the next step. Since we needed to do another therapy session in about an hour, *Magic School Bus* would be a good break for Jeremy, and it would also give me an opportunity to work.

In a few minutes Jeremy came in and mumbled a few words to me that only a mother could decipher. I managed to figure out he was asking for crackers. In therapy I had heard him speak much more distinctly the same words. I knew he was capable of more. As nicely as I could, I demanded, "Say it better."

This time Jeremy articulated plainly, "I want some crackers."

"Good, Jeremy." Standing up, I retrieved the crackers and handed him some.

In a few minutes we went to his room for my assigned timeslot for therapy.

As I positioned his table and chair, I called for him. "Jeremy, come sit down."

Looking up from playing with a new board game called Slide and Ride, he insisted, "No work, not time for work."

"No, sorry, it is time for work."

"How about Zach?" he asked hopefully.

"No," I said, tilting my head to the side.

"Heather? Jill? Heidi? Stephanie?"

I couldn't help but smile. "Sorry, you're stuck with me."

As we worked on the Vocabulary drill, he seemed bored and distracted.

"What is a cow?"

"An animal that says moo," he said.

In spite of boredom, he learned at an incredible rate each day. We needed to work harder at making therapy fun and rewarding. The Vocabulary drill especially needed to be made to be entertaining.

We encouraged Jeremy to talk, but I couldn't always understand him. Between drills he began talking, but I could only interpret a word here and there. He muttered, "Magic . . . kids . . . blood flowing . . . Frizzle." From what I could piece together, Jeremy was trying to describe the *Magic School Bus*, an animated children's science show he had watched right before my therapy session. Wow. That was good. *Magic School Bus* taught kids science in a fun way and targeted ages six to ten. And Jeremy was only four. Jeremy's brain was a gold mine that therapy had helped to open up for learning.

"Good, Jeremy. That's interesting." We needed to work on articulation badly, but I wanted to encourage his attempts.

After about a year of therapy and 1,700 hours of work, he didn't need as much prompting to get through new information. On drills he enjoyed, he sometimes had to be told the answer only once.

For *Verbal Imitation*, he was able to do about six-syllable sentences, but we needed to work up to ten-syllable sentences.

I called Jeremy to the table to introduce the *Assertiveness* drill. After we sat down, I picked up a toy dog. "Is this a cup? Say, 'No, that's a dog.'"

"No, that's a dog." His expression told me that he thought I was being silly.

He really enjoyed this drill, and when he did step four for Jill a few days later, Jill told him, "Jeremy, draw on the walls."

"No, I'm not supposed to do that."

"Cut your clothes."

"No, I'm not supposed to do that either."

I could see how a child would really need to be ready for this drill. I felt it showed how far Jeremy had progressed. After the *Assertiveness* drill we asked him questions like, "Should I pull hair?" Or a question that needed the opposite response like, "Should I follow the rules?"

By the end of that month Kristie advised me to build up to four or five peer play sessions a week. As peer play and school hours increased, the one-on-one hours decreased.

We introduced Brain Quest, an educational tool for asking questions that I purchased at the educational supply store. It consisted of a stack of cards with pictures and questions fastened together at the top. Little by little over days and weeks, we asked him questions designed for two-to-three year-olds. Then we worked on questions for age three to four and age four to five. For those questions he didn't know, we taught him to ask, "What's that?" or some appropriate question.

More and more items we introduced in therapy showed up during normal activities. Jeremy began spontaneously using words and knowledge we had taught him.

One day when Heather came over, Jeremy walked over to the window and said, "It's cloudy today." Even the *Weather* drill had contributed to his overall learning.

As winter turned into spring, Jeremy improved daily. If one of the therapists was off for a few days, they usually commented on Jeremy's progress when they returned.

As Jeremy continued to improve, instead of relaxing, I became more tense and worried about the possible outcome of therapy. It was hard to explain why I got more and more frantic for Jeremy's welfare, but I did. Would he recover? We were so close.

The tension built until I was nervous and irritable with others. I snapped at the bagger in the grocery store for no reason. Shocked, Jennifer said, "Mommy, he was just trying to be nice to you." I felt so bad that I prayed for him all the way home and told Jennifer, "Mommy was wrong. I'm sorry."

One week two therapists canceled sessions due to upcoming tests and projects in their college courses. I looked at the schedule and tried to comfort myself that I had one other person coming in the next day. Between us, I hoped we could make up for the missing hours. Did the therapists realize how close we were to seeing Jeremy through this awful problem?

The next day the phone rang, and to my dismay, the one remaining therapist announced, "Karen, I'm sorry. I can't come to work today. My boss from my other job called and needs me to come in, and I told her I would."

Anger to the point of rage boiled to the surface. "Don't I pay you enough? I really need you today. I've already had two therapists cancel." Fury spewed from every word, and I knew my annoyance could be heard.

"No, actually, you pay more. I'm sorry. I've already told my boss I'm coming, so I can't get out of it."

"Okay," I forced out through clenched teeth.

The moment the phone hit its support I burst into uncontrollable sobbing. I collapsed on the bed, my crying growing louder and louder. All the months of tension and effort to rescue Jeremy seemed to pour from my heart at the same time. It didn't make sense to react this way when Jeremy was improving so much. Who can understand how people will react during or after a crisis unless they experience a similar situation?

The therapist graciously forgave me for my outburst.

Later I confided to Kristie how I had behaved. She smiled sympathetically. "I've heard that this happens among those parents whose children make it to normal. You've been working on this a long time. You can only keep up this intense therapy so long. Also Dr. Lovaas told us to tell parents with children like Jeremy that your child may have some oddities until about fourth grade. Then they will fade too."

This bit of news encouraged me, but there was still much to overcome and more drills we had not been given yet. Though not as intense as at the beginning, the therapy would continue another year and a half, with a focus on helping Jeremy through language and social obstacles. We couldn't quit now with him so close to recovery.

At the end of the spring semester, I decided to try to get Jeremy into Jennifer's school for the next fall. We planned to enter him in half-day kindergarten for the coming school year and then full-day kindergarten the year after that. Placing him in kindergarten two years in a row had been the advice from the Early Autism Clinic, and it seemed wise. Not only did he have much to overcome, but he had a summer birthday, which made him younger than many of his classmates.

The school was a private Christian school that did not have the resources to handle special-needs children. For Jeremy to enter the school, he needed to pass a school readiness test. At that time Jeremy was four years and ten months old and had been in therapy about one year and five months. He had received approximately 2,200 hours of therapy.

The person assigned to do the testing for the preschool was a Speech Therapist, Jo Ann, who had taken time away from her job at the local hospital to do evaluations for children whose parents wished them to enter the school. She didn't know about Jeremy's history, which I felt was for the best. Her expectations would not be too high or too low. I felt she would be unbiased.

Jeremy and I met the elementary school director at the office, and we sat down across the table from Jo Ann, an attractive woman in her thirties. She greeted us then asked me, "Do you want to stay for Jeremy's test?"

"Yes, I'd really like to, if that is okay with you?"

"Yes, that's fine. You just can't help him or prompt him at anytime during the test."

I sat back and watched. I knew Jeremy's abilities, but I was surprised when he read the word *cat* from a group of words she asked if he could read. After the testing the director and the speech therapist allowed us to wait for the results. Jeremy happily played with toys.

When the director and Jo Ann walked in the room I feared the worst. The director appeared uncomfortable—her eyes shifted awkwardly down at the paper then over to me. She seemed to make a conscious effort to act natural and upbeat. Were they going to deny Jeremy admittance to the school?

The director sat down with Jeremy's test results and placed the paper in front of me. I knew Jeremy had not completed all the drills available for the ABA therapy program, so I didn't expect perfection. I braced myself for bad news.

Pointing with her pencil to the sheet with the test results, she said, "He's doing real well in his fine motor, visual motor, numbers, concepts, and body image. In fact, he's tested age level or above. However..." she stopped and cleared her voice, "he has tested from three and a half to four years old developmentally in his language and social skills. That's six to twelve months behind where he is supposed to be. Also his gross motor skills are from four months to ten months behind his age."

I just nodded my head. Words failed me. The question was would they allow Jeremy in the school? Were the results good enough?

Before I could ask any questions, she said, "He is doing well enough to enter kindergarten. But you might need to think about getting speech therapy or working at home on his language." She handed me some sheets on the developmental steps a child Jeremy's age needed.

I smiled. Would I think about helping him? Ha, if she only knew. She must have thought she was telling bad news to a mom who was hearing it for the first time. Out loud I politely thanked her. Looking down at the colored sheets of paper, I asked, "May I have these?"

"Certainly."

I could use these lists to make drills. My therapists and I could make our own drills now. We had gotten good at breaking down learning into small manageable units for Jeremy. When we saw a need, we would make up a drill and rotate it in with all the other drills.

Joy and excitement bubbled inside. What an accomplishment for Jeremy to be accepted in a regular classroom! Driving home, I couldn't wait to tell Randall.

\*\*\*

Later I shared the results of Jeremy's developmental test with Randall. "His language and social skills are only about a year behind now." I pointed to the test form and rolled my eyes. "If they only knew how far he's come. And now for the best part, read this!" I stuck the paper under his nose. Too excited to wait, I pulled it back and read it for him. "Look how well he did on the concept section. He tested two to eight months *ahead* of his age of four years and ten months. I think the concept section is one of the most important sections. It says, 'factual knowledge and reasoning skills; the ability to understand relationships; necessary for critical thinking and reasoning.'"

I stopped to take a breath. Randall smiled at me, a twinkle in his eye that reflected the joy we both felt at this improvement.

I waved the paper in the air in delight. "I'm so excited. And we're not even finished with therapy yet. He did miss a question, however, that he could easily answer in therapy a few weeks ago. I'm going to have to bring the drill back for review."

"What's that?"

"Some question to do with safety. I can't remember exactly. The answer was 'it's dangerous,' and he didn't get it. I'm really surprised."

"What else?"

"Oh, she had him echo a group of words just like the *Verbal Imitation* drill, and he could only do the first part. When she got up to what sounded like fifteen syllables, he couldn't do it. I'm not sure I can do that many syllables." I laughed. "Jeremy's up to eight syllables in therapy. Also, she wrote on the bottom, 'Jeremy was very cooperative during the test setting.' Isn't that good?" I laughed again.

Randall reached for the test and scanned the sheet. "You know? I want a day I can say, 'Let's celebrate. No more drills. No more therapy.' Will therapy ever be over?"

I too would wonder this many times in the months ahead.

# CHAPTER TWENTY:

# KINDERGARTEN—OH YES!

In the few weeks that followed the test, we attempted to work on more natural dialogue with Jeremy during therapy but had to step back and work on multiple questions and mixing easier *Conversation* drills.

I noticed in his spontaneous speech he could ask a question like, "Can I have some more crackers?" which I thought was good. But his enunciation of words still needed more work. He also needed work on more varied conversation. The good news—he no longer needed prompting on every single thing he learned.

Jeremy had advanced to some fairly complex drills like working addition problems, counting money, and telling time, but he couldn't have a conversation about what he was doing for the summer. I felt that the knowledge was in his head. We just had to help him verbalize it.

As summer progressed, the young people who had been Jeremy's therapists began to quit. Zach married and moved to another state. Jill married and stayed in the area but no longer had time to work with Jeremy. Though she didn't have time to work, her stepson became one of Jeremy's peer play friends. They are still friends today.

During summer vacation, I had a playgroup in our home once a week that we ran like a typical kindergarten class. Sympathetic friends would loan me their kids, and we shared stories, crafts, and activities with a small group of children. I picked a theme like community, space, or ponds and coordinated activities related to the topic. Keeping Jeremy active and in appropriate activities was important. I didn't want to leave any room for regression. We still had to redirect self-stimulatory behaviors on rare occasions.

At the end of the summer, two more therapists, Jessica and Stephanie, quit. One day when I had no one available to work and nothing scheduled, Jeremy asked, "Where's Zach?"

"He moved, honey." Then he began asking for each one of his other therapists by name. I had to tell him the best I could that they were gone but that Heidi would be back. Heather eventually came back to work also, but she left for a while when she got married.

\*\*\*

All summer I agonized over Jeremy being able to handle the half-day kindergarten in the fall. Heidi and Heather were the only ones working for us, and they did not have any time available in the morning to be his shadow. We decided to let him go to school on his own. I have worried about that decision so many times in the last few years. If I had it to do over again, I would have gone myself as his shadow. But at the time I felt the mommy factor would not be good for him.

Ms. White, the teacher, knew something wasn't right. She cautioned me, "Something's not right. Jeremy may have the problem my son has. My son is an A-student as long as he doesn't have to write anything. If his teachers test him orally, he's fine."

I tried to comfort her by saying, "Don't worry about it. I know Jeremy is having some problems. But we are working with him, and we plan on holding him back for another year of kindergarten." The next year we planned for Jeremy to enter the full-day kindergarten class which was a nice progression for him since he was currently in half-day kindergarten.

Since kindergarten was only mornings, in the afternoons we still continued working with him and having peer play sessions.

Jeremy made up a cute prayer at his kindergarten class. It went something like this, "Help God with the flowers and the trees." Though theologically in error, it was a precious thought and told us how far he had progressed.

One day when I picked up Jeremy at school, Ms. White walked him to the car as she did each of her students. As Jeremy crawled in the back seat and snapped his seatbelt, Ms. White leaned down to talk to me. "Jeremy talked too much in school today." She nodded her head in my direction.

"I'm sorry," I said. I looked at Jeremy and then back to Ms. White. "We'll see you tomorrow."

I drove off, and as soon as I got out of earshot I shouted, "Yes! He talked too much at school. That's wonderful." Ecstatic, I laughed, realizing it must be rare for a parent to rejoice over a child talking too much at school. Glancing in the rearview mirror, I saw Jeremy give me a funny look.

"What, Mommy?"

"Never mind, honey. I'm just happy."

\*\*\*

Another day when I picked up Jeremy after school, Ms. White greeted me and exclaimed, "Today, Jeremy said something so funny. One of the little girls started to boss everyone in class including me, and Jeremy told her, 'Anna, you're not the boss of everyone.' It was great. Totally appropriate for the situation." She laughed. She seemed encouraged by his reaction.

In spite of Ms. White's worries, Jeremy made friends at school. He even received invitations to come over and play at his friends' houses. On his own initiative he asked if he could invite one of his friends over after school. I told him, "Sure, I'll call the boy's mother." When his friend came over, Jeremy kept conversation and interaction going for about two hours without prompting. This was a major accomplishment as far as I was concerned. At such times, I wanted to declare therapy over and say, "And they lived happily ever after. The end." On the other hand, I wanted to hear it from an expert.

In an effort to put an end to therapy, I took Jeremy to my psychologist friend, Dr. Roy, who had attempted to test Jeremy in the past. The school had administered a school readiness test, but Dr. Roy would administer an IQ test. In the past, Jeremy had been unable to respond to the IQ test. This time when Jeremy was tested, the outcome was quite different. As part of the test the child is required to work several mazes. The last maze Jeremy worked was so difficult I'm not sure that I would be able to work it. His verbal IQ was 112, which is high average compared to other kids, and his performance IQ was 141, which is superior. Dr. Roy acted happier than I was at the results of the test. What a blessing to have a friend happy for my son's accomplishments!

Jeremy had some issues with his speech like irregular past tense, and some articulation issues that we had not addressed, so I continued to work with him myself.

We also worked on his gross motor skills.

We planned ahead of time for Jeremy to attend two years of kindergarten, one year to focus on academic skills and one year for social skills. Jeremy handled his first year of kindergarten well until about eight months into the school year. At that point, the curriculum and the kids took a big leap, and Jeremy couldn't make the leap with them. The teacher who had had concerns for Jeremy all year asked the director and me to discuss the options for Jeremy.

Looking at the paperwork Ms. White gave her, the director said, "From what I can tell, Jeremy will pass this school year, but it may be a source of frustration for him to move up with the class he is with. We will support you if you wish for him to go on to first grade. It's up to you."

"Thank you both, but I have already decided to hold him back for kindergarten another year."

Since Jeremy was doing so well, I decided to take him to Dr. Daniel, the child developmental specialist who had told me Jeremy was autistic when he was two and a half years old. I took some samples of Jeremy's school work, a video of him playing with other children, and a copy of the IQ test.

Jeremy and I sat together in the examination room waiting for her. I decided I would not attempt to answer for him when she asked questions, no matter what.

When she walked in the room, her gaze skipped over me and landed right on Jeremy. In return he gave her eye contact.

"Hi, Jeremy," she greeted.

"Hi," he said.

This simple exchange caused her to smile.

I leaned back in my chair, unsure if Jeremy was ready for her questions. After all the work the last two years, I thought I would be nervous. Instead I calmly listened.

Dr. Daniel asked a series of simple questions. Then she asked, "What is your favorite thing about school?"

"I like to play outside," Jeremy answered.

Dr. Daniel smiled again. "Good."

Jeremy looked bored but sat and cooperated.

Next Dr. Daniel tensed up and seemed to almost hold her breath before the next question. "Who is your best friend?"

I understood why she seemed to tense up. Few if any autistic children have friends.

"I have two good friends. Andy and Jeffrey," Jeremy said.

At this simple answer, Dr. Daniel grinned from ear to ear. Joy beamed from her countenance. If her emotions could have been charted, they would have bounced off the walls.

*He can do a lot more than this*, I thought, smiling at her reaction.

Finally she addressed me. "I wish I received good news like this every day."

I showed her the video, his school work, and the IQ test. She appeared as happy as I was about Jeremy's progress.

Her next statement had great meaning for me, and I believe it will always be a cherished memory and an important milestone of Jeremy's recovery from autism. Dr. Daniel announced, "I consider Jeremy in normal range in every developmental area."

I had told myself that hearing from a professional would be enough for me to call a halt to all the work. In spite of this significant news, I still wished for an expert who could go in and observe Jeremy with other children and tell me if they could pick him out of a group of children. This was a suggestion from the consultant. If the person could pick him out of a group of children, we could come up with drills to help him through whatever was revealing itself.

One day I received my wish. My friend Natalie came over to visit. She brought with her Annette, a friend from San Antonio whom I had never met. Natalie's two children and Jeremy played in the playroom right off the living room while we talked. After about forty-five minutes, Natalie suggested, "Karen, why don't you tell Annette about Jeremy's history?"

I gave Annette a summary of Jeremy's history.

Astonished, Annette declared, "I'm truly amazed. I'm a special ed teacher in San Antonio. I consider myself an expert in autism, and I never would have guessed it."

Wow! This was better than I had thought.

Moments like this have been repeated since that experience. Such times eased my mind, and Jeremy brought joy to Randall, Jennifer, and me.

# CHAPTER TWENTY-ONE:
# FAST FORWARD

. . . *Jeremy at age eleven*

Sitting in an audience, I watched my eleven-year-old son in his red muscle shirt and Hawaiian-style swim trunks up on the stage with other actors, smiling and singing.

In awed reflection, I silently thanked God again for the miracle of Jeremy's life. His every word was a miracle—every smile a blessing. If the crowd had known Jeremy at two years old, they would not have believed he could ever perform in front of an audience. Jeremy had become what I had hoped and prayed for—a happy, healthy child.

Jeremy delivered a funny line, and the audience laughed. He had the "surfer dude" accent down perfectly. Then Jeremy and three other actors stepped up to the microphones to sing their solos. My mind flew through the accomplishments that Jeremy's doctor believed would never happen. My heart swelled. Jeremy had a sense of humor, friends, and a normal life.

How full life was now compared to what I thought loomed ahead for us when Jeremy was two and a half. When thinking of the highs and lows of the years we worked so hard for a normal life for Jeremy, I remembered the day he came home from his second year of kindergarten and told me he was engaged to a girl at school. I didn't bother telling him kids don't get engaged at age six. Then I watched him at the Christmas party tell the girl he would miss her over the Christmas break.

I remembered asking the teacher, "Is he interacting?"

Her answer was, "He *always* interacts. And he pays attention in class better than most of the kids."

I remembered the day he came home from first grade and told me about his teacher telling the class a story about an autistic child who would fall on the floor and throw tantrums. And he calmly demonstrated it by acting it out and then stood up and continued telling me about his day.

Many times simple things have deep meaning for me: when he talks too much at bedtime—when he laughs with his friends—sits through a symphony orchestra—his sense of humor—good report cards—when he acts charming and tells me I'm the best mom in the world.

I heard at an autism conference that without ABA the recovery rate from autism is 1%. (I believe this rate may be higher now.) With ABA the probability of a normal life is 47%. When I see parents who haven't heard about ABA or can't afford it, my heart breaks.

Recently, while walking through the grocery store I saw a woman whose face looked familiar. I recognized her immediately—it was Mrs. Carson, the grandmother of the autistic boy, George. I remembered the day they came over to our house years before. George had hit the walls the whole time they visited, and he didn't speak. His inappropriate behavior had been hard on Mrs. Carson. I understood George. At that time I had been totally immersed in the world of autism, I knew some of the behaviors that could be manifested.

After a brief greeting, I asked, "How is George?"

"Not very well."

My imagination filled in the picture, but I wasn't sure I had it right. I recalled a few years ago George had gotten lost after school, trying to take the school bus home. His parents found him, but he was distraught. After that, the family started picking him up from school.

"He's eighteen now and seriously speech-impaired," said Mrs. Carson. "He gets frustrated and bangs his head. We're worried about him, but no one seems to be able to help him. ABA helps him the most, but we can't get the funds we need to implement the therapy." She talked for several more minutes outlining the problems.

What could I say to encourage this woman? Everything that came to mind seemed lame and inadequate. I mumbled, "I'm sorry to hear that."

She didn't seem to notice my discomfort. "How is your son?"

"He's doing real well. Thank you." If it had been anyone else who had known about Jeremy's problems from the past, I would have gone into more details: my son talks, has friends, goes to school unassisted, etc. I held back, not sure what to say. I didn't want her to feel bad.

"I'm glad," she commented. "We didn't get a diagnosis soon enough to get early intervention for George."

How devastating! Though I had faced some upsetting possibilities in the past and worked hard, my experience was nothing compared to what this family faced.

### ... Jeremy at age seventeen

Today, at age seventeen, Jeremy is a typical teenager with a great sense of humor. We even have to be careful not to embarrass him in front of his friends. He has and does attend school independently and without modification to the curriculum or format since Kindergarten.

I remember last year when he was invited into the National Honor Society. At the reception after the induction ceremony, he looked over at me and smiled as he visited with his friends. The boys laughed as they shared a joke. At moments like that, I remind myself of the hard work we did when he was a small child, when I had hoped, worked, and dreamed of Jeremy living a full life. And here the dream was being lived out in the heart and mind of my son Jeremy.

I'm so thankful for God's help. My husband and I found the therapy that would reach our son amid the barrage of therapy approaches. In the process of helping our son, every resource we had available was stretched to the max: our marriage, our finances, our time, and our energies. My husband Randall worked so hard to earn the income we needed while I put my time and energy into Jeremy's therapy. We needed every person, every dime, and every word of encouragement to be successful. I have never worked so hard or stretched myself so much.

A recent picture of my teenage son in a tuxedo for his senior class portrait reflects a handsome, healthy young man. The smile on his face and the intelligence in his eyes speak of a developmentally whole person. I remember the day Jeremy was born, when I held him in my arms with such hope and promise in my heart for a bright future for my son. With God's help, hope has been restored. Jeremy is a happy, well-adjusted person, a contributor to our society. He does everything from driving a car to dating girls. He is college bound and has been accepted at the college of his choice.

Studies have verified that ABA conducted under proper conditions will bring some autistic children to normal functioning. But for me, Jeremy's recovery will always be a miracle.

## Notes to the Reader from Three of Jeremy's Therapists

Fall of 2009

**Heather**: My memories of Jeremy go back more than 15 years. Jeremy was a wide-eyed, cute toddler and I was a college student who happened on an interesting job doing ABA therapy. I was such a rookie in the world of ABA, but learned quickly and loved every second of my job with Jeremy and his precious family. I had no idea that over the next four years, I would be blessed to witness a child who had few communication skills grow into a boy who would tenaciously do 36 hours of therapy a week, gain language, engage with friends, giggle at silly songs, and eventually lose his diagnosis of autism. What a privilege!

I am a mom now to four children, a couple of them having special needs of their own. As my family has grown, I have often thought about Jeremy and how he must be doing. I have considered how different of a therapist I would be today, understanding a little better the desperation and urgency to have my children healthy and "normal" (whatever normal is!).

I can hardly believe that Jeremy is a six-foot-tall senior in high school, graduating a year early. I am so excited for him and can't wait to hear how God continues to work and bless in his life.   ~**Heather**

\*\*\*

**Heidi**: Hello my name is Heidi! And I would like to share a little from my perspective on working on such an awesome mission—which is how I felt working with Jeremy—like I was on a mission to help reclaim his life.  I was part of his life for approximately three years. Every day in the beginning was both mentally and physically draining for me just knowing the importance of my role.  Some days came with either tears of joy or tears of frustration.  Joy when a milestone was reached and frustration when we just didn't get as far as we wanted. But as the days went by, we made huge strides in reclaiming his life.  Just knowing I had a part in this mission is a ***blessing***. It is indescribable by words, but I can tell you I would not have missed it for anything!  There is ***hope!*** ~**Heidi**

\*\*\*

**Zach**: Honestly, when I agreed to work with Jeremy, it was one of the most frightening undertakings I had ever engaged in.  I was afraid—afraid that we would fail—afraid that this beautiful child would remain locked inside of himself—and afraid that this determined, faithful, and loving family would never know the joy of really knowing their son.

But the beauty of "lost causes" is that they drive us to quit or they drive us to God. And this family was not the quitting type. So we all embraced the program of therapy, but more importantly, we all agreed to pray for Jeremy.

I, for one, needed the grace and wisdom of God. How do you reach a child who won't tell you how to reach him? It was such a challenge to learn what he would respond to.

One day, out of desperation, I tickled him as a reward for completing a particularly distasteful task. To my surprise, it worked! The more I tickled, the better he performed, and the more he learned.

A few months later I arrived for a session to find Jeremy in the dining room finishing up lunch. When he saw me he turned, raised his hands, and said "tickle?" To me, that little word was like the sight of Lazarus stepping out of the tomb. As far as I know, it was the first time he'd ever asked for anything in his life. I knew then that God was listening and that Jeremy had his attention. **~Zach**

\*\*\*

## Note to the Reader from Jeremy's Dad

When most parents have toddlers, they are worried about saving money for college. But for us, we worried about financing therapy so Jeremy could get into the first grade—paying the equivalent of a college education in therapy to get him there. The rescue of Jeremy was difficult, intense, and very testing. Only small, incremental positive changes encouraged us to continue, which necessitated radical priorities which tested us for several years. These priorities included the condition of our house and cars and monetary sacrifices. But it was worth it. The benefits of a whole, healthy, smart and social son made it all worth every penny. I can tease him, and he will retaliate and interact with clever humor back to me. Now my wife and I get to worry about paying for his college. ~**Randall**

\*\*\*

## Note to the Reader from my Daughter Jennifer, Jeremy's Sister

I had a wish. I remember when I was about 3 ½ years old and wished for a younger sibling. I was an only child, and my friends at preschool all had brothers or sisters. I debated for a while whether I wanted a brother or a sister, and I decided a brother would be best so that Dad would not be alone in a house full of girls.

Not understanding what it takes to have a baby, I asked my parents for a brother. Lucky for me, they wanted another child, and lucky for them they had Jeremy, a boy.

When he came home from the hospital, I remember how red and scrawny he was and how much he SLEPT! I wanted to play with him right off, and I was perplexed that Jeremy was sleeping when I woke up in the morning and when I got home. To test my patience even more, Mom said he was too little to play. . . which I didn't understand at the time. And I would have to wait until Jeremy grew up some.

So I waited. But when Jeremy got older, about two years old, I could tell Mom and Dad were concerned. I noticed it too: Jeremy wasn't talking like other children, he didn't respond when we talked to him, and sometimes he would do this weird thing with his eyes and flap his hands. I didn't realize how serious it was. Mom and Dad sat me down and told me Jeremy had autism, and it was going to take intensive therapy for him to get well. I can't remember if they verbally told me they wouldn't be able to spend as much time with me, or if they tried to tell me the therapy was for my benefit too, since I would be Jeremy's guardian when my parents died. . . whatever the case, I never felt neglected, and I was never jealous of Jeremy, and the time I did get with my parents felt more than enough. And whether it was the lack of understanding of a six year old of the gravity of the situation or the fact that God just gave me assurance, I had no doubt that Jeremy could recover. From my silly child perspective, I thought therapy would be great since Jeremy would be able to talk by the end of it AND be able to really play.

In the meantime, I forced Jeremy to play with me despite his unresponsiveness. . . I tied a rope to both of our waists and dragged him with me around the house so we could play together. It was quite effective, but it was difficult for me to tie the rope around him sometimes, so therapy was the real cure to our playtime and allowed us to really have a true relationship.

Once the therapy got into full swing, Jeremy worked hard and made great, fast progress. I remember coming home from school, and the therapists my parents hired were working with him. The funny thing was—I wanted to be the therapists' friend too. I was a little hurt when I couldn't sit in on the therapy sessions sometimes. Looking back on it now though, I was not the reason the therapists were at my house; they were there for Jeremy. And if my not being in the room during the session helped, it was well worth it.

One thing that bugs me about Jeremy's past struggle is when we run into someone from our past that knew of Jeremy's former condition and they treat him differently. It makes me angry. Can't they see that he is normal? Don't they know that therapy can completely take away and cure the effects of autism? Don't they know that he is in the National Honor Society at school, and he has plans to go to college, get a career, and have a normal life? He asks girls out, he has friends, and he is kinder and smarter than "normal" boys in his class. I suppose it's the big sister in me that gets angry, but I want to shake them and speak my mind.

Today Jeremy and I are very close. I forget he had autism. Even when people say "autism", I don't connect it with Jeremy, even though I know what autism is, because Jeremy is SO normal. He is one of my favorite people in the whole wide world. He teases me, jokes with me, and plays games with me (even still at 17 and 21 years old). At six-feet tall, he'll even be my "bodyguard" when I go places at night. I still drag him places, but I don't need a rope anymore. Wishes… lucky for me, my younger brother was a wish that exceeded my dreams. **~Jennifer**

# APPENDIX

## Thoughts about Hope, Success, and Older Children in Therapy

I hope you have learned from my story—not just from my successes but from my failures. I write to you in a manner as if you were my sister or brother. I want you to have information and wisdom. I want you to be successful. My deepest desire is for as many as possible to get help. In the past, autism was considered a "lifelong, incapacitating, incurable" condition, but I strongly believe there is hope.

If you are anything like my husband and me, you have discovered that you must take ownership of your child's care. The likelihood of someone like Anne Sullivan coming along will probably not happen for any of us.

You may ask—what if it is too hard to implement therapy—not enough money, my child is too old, etc.? My thought is that you can glean from ABA principles what you can—for instance—I know a parent who told me, "I don't have the money to implement ABA therapy, but I studied the therapy approach and was able to teach my son how to answer a yes/no question using ABA therapy."

How about George's family, the eighteen-year-old autistic man, whose family found that George benefited most from ABA? The principles of the therapy were modified to his level of development and provided him a positive learning environment.

Applied Behavioral Analysis – Lovaas style is the main key that brought Jeremy to a place that he caught up academically and socially with other children his age, but I understand there are many other successful groups who offer ABA services. You can do the research and find a group that best fits your child's needs. The studies say that 47% of the autistic children who meet the set criteria of the study can become indistinguishable from their peers with an ABA program—started young enough, with 40 hours per week, etc. (Sallows et al, 2005).

I remember during our years of therapy I asked, will my child be in the 47% or not? This question came up often in discussions with other parents of young autistic children. We knew there were about 1% of the autistic children who receive ABA therapy who did not do well.

Also, what happens to the other 52%—that mid-range group that didn't fall in the 47% or the 1%? I saw a film of a child (Anderson, 1988) who was in the study in the '80s and received intense ABA therapy program and fell in the mid-range group. In my opinion, this young man appeared to me to be considerably improved compared to many others with autism. I remember running our therapy program, taking consolation in this fact. In addition, I heard that the young man in the original study, who represented the 1%, worked at McDonalds as an adult. Considering the most severe cases of autism are institutionalized—this is a significant improvement over those who do not have intense ABA treatment as young children.

## Educate Yourself

**1. Learn from the people who have researched and experienced autism before you. Study the right books.** (See suggested reading list.) Pick the brains of parents and professionals who are doing the therapy right. If you meet someone whose child is not making any progress for some reason, learn what you can and go on with your program. You can't afford to get sidetracked into wrong therapy approaches or those that don't understand how to run an effective ABA program. Before we ran the program for our son, we visited several workshops for other children and came away wiser. I remember worrying—what if all this work is in vain? I would comfort myself by telling myself, at least I know that I would have tried the best therapy approach available and put forth the effort. It is better than living with regret.

**2. What about using the Public School system?** Before we started ABA, my son was in a special-needs preschool class offered by the public school system. I soon discovered they never gave him one-on-one attention. Even the promise of once-a-week speech therapy never materialized. When I asked why they said, "No problem—he is in group speech therapy." I'm sure compared to what they are up against and the number of children they need to see, this is acceptable. But for my son, this just wasn't enough. Autistic children need one-on-one therapy and a lot of it. Public school teachers will rarely go along with this. I can hear them say now, "But we don't want your son to be dependent on anyone." I realized they missed the idea completely when they say this. They don't understand. Though well-meaning, using public school is like using the proverbial teacup to put out a forest fire. It will rarely, if ever, be enough to overcome autism or make important strides.

My son received thousands of hours of one-on-one therapy, and he never became dependent on any of his therapists. What did happen? Jeremy learned what he needed to learn and began to interact and form friendships.

**3. Look for what is successful.** If I had to do therapy over again, I would definitely run an ABA program. I would also provide Jeremy with nutritional help—vitamins and test for food allergies. For some children, this is huge, and I believe it helped Jeremy learn. Whatever is reasonable, successful, and financially feasible, go for it. If you are like me, anything that helps your child is worth it.

## Basic Therapy Concepts

Therapy seems so simple when you watch it being done, but there is a whole lot more to it than meets the eye. For example, before we had a consultant, I had watched therapy and read about the therapy but was a total failure at using positive reinforcements when needed. Having correct ways to reinforce correct behavior was critical in Jeremy's program. We had taught him information like action verbs and following simple instructions before we had a consultant, but without the correct approach, we were still seeing hand-flapping and other autistic behaviors. Knowledge was important for Jeremy, but if he had knowledge yet failed to be disciplined and focused enough to use that information, we were failing him—he was still in an isolated world of autism. Once we got Jeremy's program going in the right direction, hand-flapping, the odd way he shifted his eyes, and other autistic behaviors faded. These behaviors faded without addressing them directly. In other words, if he was flapping his hands during therapy, we said, "Hands quiet," and if necessary, we placed his hands flat on the table. Then we started immediately into teaching him one of his drills. As appropriate behavior and knowledge took over in Jeremy's life, autistic behavior disappeared.

## Definitions / Glossary

Therapy terms such as SD (Discriminative Stimulus), mass trialing, reinforcing stimulus, and many other terms are in the material when studying Behavioral Intervention. (ABA and Behavioral Intervention are the same.) I will simplify terms as much as possible. Progression of drills, knowledge, and the overall program for ABA is happening all at once in an ABA program. For instance, there is progression within one drill, and there is a progression for the overall drill. And there is progression of the whole program.

The following is not meant to be a complete guide, but a little information to get you started in the right direction.

**Autism**—according to The Hope Institute for Children and Families on the website, www.theautismprogram.org, the answer to the question "what is autism?" is as follows—"Autism Spectrum Disorders (ASDs) are a group of neurologically-based developmental disabilities. Scientists do not know exactly what causes the problem. ASDs can impact a person's functioning across a wide range, from very mild to severe. Individuals with ASD are not different in appearance, but they may communicate, interact, behave and learn in ways that are different from typical peers."

**Applied Behavior Analysis (or Behavioral Intervention)**—is defined by The Hope Institute for Children and Families (www.theautismprogram.org) as "an intensive, structured teaching program. Lessons to be taught are broken down to their simplest elements. Children are presented with a stimulus through repeated trials. Positive reinforcement is used to reward correct responses and behaviors, and incorrect responses are ignored."

**Discrete trial**—is a three-part teaching process for making learning clear and concise. It consists of the instruction by the therapist (SD), and the response by the child (R) and the reward/consequence (SR). (See the three steps defined—SD, R, SR)

**Drill (or Program)**—is a term normally used for the individual learning exercise used to teach a child. Examples of drills are exercises in areas such as verbs, storytelling, conversation, games, and social interaction. The sheet for a drill normally contains the instruction or question to ask the child, the expected response, the instructions and the progression of the drill. There are literally hundreds of drills available through an ABA consultant.

**MT (Mass trials)**—the term means how you introduce a new item or reintroduce an item. If you introduce the label for an apple, you say, "What is this? Say, 'apple.'" In other words, a mass trial always has the answer paired with the instruction or question.

**PDD (Pervasive Development Disorder)**—is a diagnosis giving children who either have a less severe case of autism or who have under eight behavioral symptoms of autism. (Gerlach, 1996, p. 5)

**Probe**—is to determine if a child knows the answer to a particular item in a drill. For example, if we were introducing the Labeling drill, we would sit him down to see if he could identify the items we were targeting. If not, the item(s) were introduced into his program.

**Prompt**—is when you give the answer or hint to the answer to the SD. Prompts should be faded.

**R (Response)**—your child's response to the SD whether a non-verbal, verbal, or action. If your child does not respond, that is considered an incorrect response.

**Self-Stimulation Behaviors** (or **stimming**, the slang word for self-stimulatory behavior)—are repetitive body movements or repetitive movement of objects such as head banging, rocking, spinning the body, gazing at lights, or flapping hands. All are common behaviors in autistic individuals.

**SD (Discriminative Stimulus)**—is the question, statement, or instruction to your child that you expect a response. An example of a SD—"What is your name?" or "Clap your hands." (Don't ask me why they didn't call it DS. Discriminative Stimulus is SD in the literature on Behavioral Intervention.)

**SR (Reinforcing stimulus)**—is the consequence of a child's response. If the child is correct, give an enjoyable reward—verbal praise, a hug, etc. If your child gives an incorrect response, normally respond with an informational no or silence. Hopefully, rewards correspond with how hard the child is working.

**Studies on Applied Behavior Analysis (ABA) / Behavioral Intervention**—See http://www.lovaas.com/research.php. There have been several studies on the effectiveness of ABA.

## Sample Reward List

(Must be what is rewarding to each individual child—and can change as the program progresses.)
1. Verbal praise
2. Bubbles
3. Balloons
4. Noisemaker
5. A hug
6. Food (Food is a controversial reward to use. Some find it demeaning. Others fear using food as a reward can lead to an eating-disorder. In our case, food was a distraction for Jeremy, so we stopped using food. However, I did visit a workshop where this worked well for a child. He received a couple of M&Ms after 5-7 SDs.)

APPENDIX

## Sample "Wake Up" List

(Must be geared to child.)
  1. Have Superman action figure give the SD
  2. Blow a whistle
  3. Pat head then rub noses
  4. Hook thumbs together into a pretend butterfly, fly to the child's ribcage and tickle child
  5. Use arms to make a T-Rex motion, making sound-effects
  6. Sing and act-out Eitsy-Bitsy Spider song


## Hiring

**Advertise for therapist**. It is difficult to hire enough good people to work as therapists, so you will have to come up with resourceful ways to find people you can trust to teach your child. Ideas: Post signs on bulletin boards near the education and psychology departments at the local community college and local university. Call the head of the department to see if they can announce your need of employees to their classes. Write up something the professor can read off a paper. Remember you will interview carefully and call for references. Idea for signs: create a sign with a colorful graphic (mine had A-B-Cs graphics) and the following information: (sample)

### Tutor Job
Opening to teach one-on-one
a 3-year-old child diagnosed with autism.
Great experience for special ed or psychology majors.
Training will be provided.
Call (your name here) at ___-___.   $_.__ an hour
Flexible hours – in 2 hour blocks

At the bottom of the sign, tape a strip with your first name and number multiple times so that interested students can tear off the number. Also, put your ad in with the student employment office at the university as well. For us, we received more responses from the bulletin board ads, but even if you receive interest from one important person, it is worth the effort.


## Paperwork

### Payroll Taxes, Employee Paperwork, and Payroll Organization

During our time of hiring, I researched what to do about payroll taxes and learned how to file all the necessary reports. It turned out that none of our employees made enough money to warrant the filing. The government returned our information and money. Check with a CPA regarding the current requirements or IRS publications 926 has information for how to file for household employees.

After you hire someone, make a folder with their name on it. Keep inside their folder a form for them to sign in and out when they work. Set up a table in the kitchen or dining room or convenient room near where the therapist will be. The area can have the work schedule for the week, their folder for signing in, and the therapy book. (More on the therapy book later.)

### More on Payroll Organization

Have a regular payday if possible. Write on each employee's time sheet what you are paying along with the calculations and check number. Most of the time, I had an agreement with the person when I would pay. For instance, bi-monthly I would sit down after a therapy session and write them a check. Another option is to place the check in an envelope and put it in their folder so that they can receive their check the next time they work. However, I never paid for future hours.

If you pay your employees different rates, be sure to find a way to keep the folders private. I'd like to think that no one would look, but there were rare moments that our therapists had the opportunity to look. Since everyone knew each other's name, and they knew the pay scale, there was nothing confidential. I had an understanding with each person that freshmen received a set amount and for each grade level slightly more. I had a college graduate and a Ph.D. student that received more pay, but no one seemed to be concerned about the low pay. The money mainly kept everyone accountable to one another. Most knew I was doing my best.

## Interviewing

When you set up an interview, provide a professional atmosphere as much as possible in spite of the fact that you meet in your home. Have them fill out an application—ask for name, address, phone number, available time slots to work, references, work experience, etc. Even knowing unrelated work references are helpful. If you find out someone is faithful to previous jobs, this is a good sign. You have probably found someone who will take the job seriously.

Create a document on your computer that you can use for interviews so that you can reprint as many times as you need it. During the interview, educate the applicant on what autism is and what you are trying to accomplish—that you hope to rescue your child from autism, what ABA is, etc. Make sure and explain what will be expected of them including the commitments for workshops. Observing their reaction may help you know if they are truly interested in the job. Analyze the person to discover whether you can trust him or her with your child. You will be calling on references, but trust your instincts as well. Also, can this person be fun and make therapy motivating and entertaining?

## Schedules

When therapy first began for Jeremy, I scheduled 36 hours a week. If I had it to do over again, I believe I would schedule the full 40 hours as the consultant suggested. Sometimes the therapists were unable to work their hours in which case Jeremy didn't always receive the hours he needed if I was unable to fill the time myself. Since the time we ran Jeremy's therapy program, I read about a study that said that autistic children who received 15-25 hours of therapy were helped but did not accomplish the significant gains as the group that received 40 hours a week (Howard et al., 2005). So the amount of time worked is important.

As stated before, we worked six days a week, six hours a day in two hour sessions. I tried to get a commitment from each person on what hours they had available to work. As much as I would have liked the schedule to be the same each week, it didn't happen that way. I found myself filling the schedule each week. Usually about two or three people were consistent with their hours and this helped, but I had to fill the open hours as well. So when someone came in to work, I verified their work schedule for the next week and asked if they could fill empty therapy slots. For my personal therapy work hours, I filled about six hours a week. This was purposely a low amount of hours for several reasons—sometimes I filled hours when someone canceled at the last minute—I acted as my own lead therapist, so I was busy lining up props for drills, scheduling, planning, hiring, etc. I found I would burnout easily because when therapy was not scheduled I needed to make sure Jeremy did not sit around doing things that fed autistic behaviors. For the three-to-five-p.m. time slot, I always tried to fill this time slot with others. This was the time slot I would pick up Jennifer from school, have the opportunity to spend a little time with her, and cook dinner for the evening. I remember meeting other mothers who spent up to twenty hours a week of therapy time with their child. I found this impossible for myself. With the unofficial time with Jeremy, it was already a 24/7 kind of effort. I found myself exhausted or near tears if I didn't watch myself. We are all built differently, and I discovered quickly how many hours I could handle.

A note here to parents that do not make good therapists: That is okay—don't be hard on yourself. I heard this is common. Not everyone has what it takes to work with their child for a number of reasons. Most of all the emotional involvement makes it very difficult to provide the discipline needed to be a therapist. If this is the case, leave it to your therapists to run your program. Usually one of your therapists will stand out as someone who can run the program. In this case, pay the person a little more than the rest and have them be your lead therapist.

Having people constantly in and out of our house was a bit of a strain at times—not bad, but sometimes challenging. I'm a terrible housekeeper, and I had to straighten our house multiple times each day. Sometimes I forgot to check the therapy room to make sure it was cleaned up for the next person. This was hard on the next therapist. I tried to implement a rule that each person had to leave the room in as good a shape as they found it, but this was difficult to enforce. If I had to hire now, I would spell this out during the interview process.

## Meetings

I tried having employee meetings weekly. This was a good time to inspire everyone, discuss drills and strategies, and help new therapists, etc. Often we brought Jeremy in to illustrate how to implement a new drill. Between meetings and occasionally in place of meetings, I would brief therapists for the first few minutes after they arrived for work. I also left Post-its with instructions when needed in the therapy book to make sure each person kept on task. At workshops, the consultant trained everyone on how to progress with a drill—from the introduction of a new item to the review of an item. I found that not everyone was good at implementing the progression of items. So, I kept tabs on the drills. Some therapists were good at this and others were not, so I checked in on the drills daily.

## Workshops

Workshops were always a boost to our program with Jeremy. I would find out what weekends the therapists had available time and try to schedule the workshops for the best time for everyone. I made sure everyone knew how important this was to helping Jeremy and that it was a high priority. Besides scheduling a workshop with the consultant, I made reservations at a local hotel for her to stay and planned food for during the workshop. Normally, her travel agent scheduled the flight and I would pay by credit card over the phone.

I paid each therapist their hourly rate for all the hours they were at the workshop and fed everyone their lunch meals. Except for the first workshop that lasted three days, we had two-day workshops approximately every three months for Jeremy on Saturday and Sunday—this provided a time when most people would be free to come. In spite of the fact that I try not to miss church unless I am ill or there is an emergency—I felt like having workshops for Jeremy fell into a category of an emergency. I announced to all my therapists and church family that we would be filling 8am to 5pm on both Saturday and Sunday which caused us to miss church. Everyone was very gracious and understanding.

Also before each workshop, I found that if I made sure each therapist was as well-trained as possible, it saved time at workshops and helped us make the most of the time we had with the consultant. Having a workshop was an expensive undertaking, and I wanted to make the most of it. I encouraged the therapists to ask questions, but if I knew the answer, I might as well answer questions beforehand. Resolving unanswered issues as much as possible helped at workshops. I also found out that I had to hire a babysitter for workshops. As Jeremy progressed and improved, he no longer kept to himself. He wanted to interact with the therapists. If I didn't hire someone to give him snacks and keep him entertained, he was in the workshop much of the time trying to get our attention. As much as that was a good sign of his healing, we needed to keep with the task at hand. Though, he was called in to work periodically.

For some of our workshops, we invited some parents from our autism support group who came to observe. I made it clear to them and to any visitors who came, not to hold up the progression of a workshop with talking. They were welcomed to talk or ask questions if there was a lull or at mealtime, but I made it clear that the consultant had the floor and this was about Jeremy. Everyone received this amiably and was very kind. I'm normally a mild-mannered soul, but my son's life was at stake. This cause alone turned me into a mother bear protecting her young.

## Therapy and Time Issues

During our time of running what I call a mega-therapy program for our son, my husband and I didn't have a life it seemed. We did good to go to church on Sunday and talk to our family and friends occasionally. If you run a therapy program, don't be too hard on yourself. This is a once in a lifetime opportunity to make a lasting impact on your child's life. My sisters used to be shocked at how little I was able to talk to them during those months of therapy and remind me of those days sometimes when we visit. Inform your family and friends that this time is temporary. When you get to the end of the drills, you can phase back into a more normal schedule. No matter how well your child is doing, he/she may require some type of review therapy depending on how well the outcome.

## Babysitting Issues

I never used a therapist as a babysitter unless I paid the person extra and had an understanding with her first. My husband and I always changed diapers and did not expect this from the therapists. Our therapists were not babysitters—they were therapists.

## Recordkeeping for Therapy

Documentation is an important part of therapy. It helps in an ABA program to: measure progress, know what to introduce, know what/when to review an item, etc. Recordkeeping helps you and your therapists identify what current drills are active and the item within the drill that is active. How to record drills and their progress was such a mystery to me, but it ended up being an easy process. The recordkeeping therapy book consisted of—a three-inch binder, notebook paper, and dividers. In the notebook was the list of current programs, a behavior section and sections for each active drill.

Current program checklist: This form includes the form name on the top of the page, and the table with about twenty-five rows and eight columns wide. The column headings are labeled: first column is the name of the drill. Column two through seven are the days of the week abbreviated—M,T,W,T,F,S,S. The therapists mark a tally for each time a drill is worked for any particular day. I have included a sample checklist here.

| Program Name | M | T | W | T | F | S | S |
|---|---|---|---|---|---|---|---|
| What's Missing? | III | | | | | | |
| Categories | II | | | | | | |
| Occupations | III | | | | | | |
| (Add as many rows as needed, with blank lines for changes) | | | | | | | |

So in the chart, the three tally marks for What's Missing and Occupations mean that these two programs were done three times on Monday, and the Categories program was done twice on Monday.

**Behavior section:** At the end of a therapy session, the therapist wrote in this section regarding Jeremy's behavior in free format style. The therapist wrote the date, their name, and a short paragraph regarding behavior that day. The next person skipped a line and continued following with the same format.

**Program sections:** Normally there were about fifteen active programs at any given time. We placed fifteen dividers with the name of the drill on each tab. Within each section was the instruction sheet, a checklist of items to be mastered and blank paper behind that. The instruction sheet included the SD, expected response, and usually the progression of the drill.

When a therapist arrived, they signed in, took the therapy book and Jeremy to the therapy room. Note here: Some parents have closed-circuit TV or videotaping in therapy sessions—with the therapists' knowledge, of course. You may choose to do this to make sure drills are executed correctly, etc.

Back to the workflow of a therapy session—opening the book, the therapist would turn the page to the first drill or the place the last person left off. The first page of the section had instructions on how to implement the drill and many times the next step or steps to that drill. The next pages were blank and were used to document the progress. The column headings were: date, therapist name, item we worked on, and results. Here is an example of documentation for the drill behind the tab, "Where…?" drill:

| Date | Therapist | Item (Question/Statement) | Results |
|------|-----------|---------------------------|---------|
| 2/20 | Karen | Where do you keep milk? | w/o prompt 2/3 |

The number of times asked was the bottom number, and the number of times he responded correctly was the top number. Sometimes under the line was a comment needed for the next person. We added words or codes we all understood, for instance: MT for mass trial which means we introduced something for the first time and the next person might need to prompt. If the expected response wasn't written with the question, it was on the drill instruction sheet. Skimming through the drills, I could quickly tell what he had mastered and what needed work. Some drills had a summary sheet in the front of the section where we checked off what he had mastered.

Also, we might have a group of questions we needed to find out if he knew the answer. We would write "probe" next to the question and what the results were. Probing meant we found out what he knew. If he didn't know the information, we did not correct him during a probe because he was not expected to know the answer yet. However, if he did know the answer, it was good to reward him. Any unknown items were mass trialed at a later time.

We eventually had review books we worked from in addition to the current drills. This book used the same format as the regular therapy book. We came up with ways to rotate review items to make sure he remembered previously taught information. At times, we had to bring back an item to work with him.

## Peer Play

When your child has met all the prerequisites for peer play, there are goals to strive for in this program.

### Goals
Respond to peer when peer initiates interaction
Build conversation
Turn taking
Make sure peer has fun and wants to come back

Games
Imaginary play
Therapist starts play and then fades out (*at the beginning, therapist participates)

## Items to Take Note of on Peer Sheet Documentation
Does child follow directions?
Does child talk during activities?
Does child initiate activities with peer?
Was there any inappropriate behavior or socially unacceptable behavior?
Was child hyper or zoned out?
Is there an area that needs work that we need to create a drill?

Thought: Create a document your therapist can work with during peer play sessions. Here is a sample document:

## Peer Play Activity List
Therapist Name _____
Peer's Name _____
Date _____

## Mock Pre-School
Circle Time
Non Verbal Imitation
Statement/Statement
If/Then
Story Time
Book Questions
Songs
Other _____

## Pretend
Super Boy
Cars/Racing or Train
Doll House (People)

Fire Truck/Save babies
School
Camping Trip
Birthday Party
Three Bears Story
Other _____

**Games**
Take turns working a twenty-five piece puzzle
Hi Ho Cherrio
Animal Dominoes
Maisy Game
Barnyard Bingo
Ring Around the Rosies
Hide and Seek
Follow the Leader
Duck Duck Goose
Red Light/Green Light
Memory game
London Bridges
Outside Play (play ball, sidewalk chalk, etc.)
Legos
Big Blocks
Peanut Panic
Fanatic Ants
KooKooNauts
Don't Wake Daddy
Other _____

Did the Peer have fun? _____

    I fit as much as possible on one page sheet using two columns for ease of use for the therapists. I also listed the goals on the form as well, along with codes to help them document the session. The therapist would circle the activities or fill in the blank. Also, the therapist would write notes on areas to work on.

At the end of a peer play session, I let Jeremy and his friend pick a small inexpensive toy out of a box I kept full of fun items. This was reinforcing for the kids and hopefully helped cause peers to want to come back. Sometimes I provided snack time which was fun, and also provided an opportunity to work on conversation. For instance, I might start talking about going to McDonalds and what I ate which was a drill for Jeremy.

## Post Therapy:  Success and Depression

Though therapy was successful beyond what I thought possible, after therapy was over, I was depressed. I know this is hard to believe and though I was extremely thankful for Jeremy's healing, I was depressed none the less. It seems like a contradiction, but I've been told that this can be typical of someone who has overcome a difficult obstacle. I held things together during therapy, but when therapy was over, it was a major adjustment. In hindsight, it sounds ungrateful. We had received our miracle. I talked to a professional later that said I probably had an adjustment disorder.

I have added this section for those who may find it difficult to ease back into a more normal routine after mega-therapy is over. Besides being depressed, I remember being so burned-out I thought I would never have another ambition again. I just went through the motions of life, but without the heart and energy of the past. It took years to feel like my old self. During that time period, others never would have suspected, but I was different. Hopefully, you find no difficulties in the transition from mega-therapy to normal life.

For me, the time of depression was relatively short-lived, but the burned-out state lasted for about five years and only time seemed to heal. If you go through any of these feelings, I hope this warning helps you prepare yourself mentally. If you find your depression is prolonged, consult a doctor or professional.

## Hope and Final Words of Encouragement

My sincere prayer is that a helpful and encouraging atmosphere be provided for those seeking to rescue their children diagnosed with autism. The barrage of facts and information is as overwhelming as ever. However, as the most successful treatment approaches that helped Jeremy came into focus for us, I feel that the right treatment(s) can come into focus for others as well. Don't procrastinate—start now, even if you can only do one small thing each day or each week. I sincerely hope that this book will lighten your load. I hope my journey has helped clear the way for others so there are fewer obstacles to face. If you haven't already done so, consider asking God to walk with you on this journey. He is a faithful Friend and provides strength and help. May God grant the strength and purpose to follow-through on the task of helping our children.

Blessings,

*Karen*

## Helpful Links & More Information on Autistic Behaviors, Studies, etc.

www.aLifetoRescue.com, my website for links and information
www.lovaas.com, Lovaas Institute for Early Invention
www.autism.com, Autism Research Institute

# Reading List

Teaching Individuals with Developmental Delays: Basic Intervention Techniques by O. Ivar Lovaas

Behavioral Intervention for Young Children with Autism: A Manual for Parents and Professionals, by Catherine Maurice, Gina Green, Stephen C. Luce

Making a Difference: ABA for Autism, by Catherine Maurice, Gina Green, Richard M. Foxx

Let Me Hear Your Voice, by Catherine Maurice

ABA for Autism for Young Children with Autism, Edited by Catherine Maurice

Meer 1: Manual of Exercises for Expressive Reasoning by Linda Zachman, Mark Barrett, Rosemary Huisingh, Carolyn Blagden, Jane Orman

For information on Audio Integration training—see www.vision-audio.com and the book The Sound of a Miracle by Annabel Stehli. Unfortunately, I could not tell any difference in Jeremy's behavior or skills after implementing audio integration training, but wanted to provide this information for those who feel it will help their child.

Current locations and contact information for clinics that help implementing an Applied Behavioral Analysis—Lovaas Style program can be found on the website www.lovaas.com. Wisconsin Early Autism Project provided workshops in Texas when we needed a clinic, but at the printing of this book, Wisconsin does not provide services to Texas. Those interested will need to check the website for information on the location serving your area. There are other excellent ABA groups. Be sure to research.

# References

Anderson, E. L. (Producer). (1988). Behavioral treatment of autistic children with o. ivar [Videocassette]. (Currently available at http://store.behavior.org/)

Centerwall, W. R. (June 1989). An introduction to your child who has autism [Brochure]. Redmond, Washington: Medic Publishing Co.

Gerlach, E. K. (1996/2003). Autism treatment guide (Rev Edition/3rd ed.). Eugene, Oregon: Four Leaf Press.

Howard, J. S., Sparkman, C. R., Cohen, H. G., Green, G., & Stanislaw, H. (2005). A comparison of intensive behavior analytic and eclectic treatments for young children with autism. Research in Developmental Disabilities, 26, 359-383.

Lovaas, O. I. (1981). Teaching developmentally disabled children: The me book. Austin, TX: Pro-Ed.

Lovaas, O. I. (1987). Behavioral treatment and normal educational and intellectual functioning in young autistic children. Journal of Consulting and Clinical Psychology, 55, 3-9. (Newer studies confirm these findings (Sallows & Graupner, 2005). Also see http://www.lovaas.com/research.php)

McEachin, J. J., Smith, T., & Lovaas, O. I. (1993). Long-term outcome for children with autism who received early intensive behavioral treatment. American Journal of Mental Retardation, 97(4), 359-372.

Rimland, B., & Kanner, M. L. (January 1964). Infantile autism: the syndrome and its implications for a neural theory of behavior. Upper Saddle River, New Jersey: Prentice Hall.

Sallows, G. O., & Graupner, T. D. (2005). Intensive behavioral treatment for children with autism: Four-year outcome and predictors. American Journal of Mental Retardation, 110(6), 417-438.

## About the Author

Karen Michelle Graham is a wife and mother of two children, a 22-year-old daughter, Jennifer, and a 17-year-old son, Jeremy. Karen received a Bachelor of Arts in Business Management, worked as a computer programmer for fourteen years, and is currently a writer and speaker. Her desire is to provide help and information to other parents, just as she has been helped.

### For more information or to order books, eBooks, or audiobooks, visit:

www.aLifetoRescue.com

### To schedule Karen for a speaking engagement, e-mail:

speak@aLifetoRescue.com

CPSIA information can be obtained
at www.ICGtesting.com
Printed in the USA
LVOW12s1953101017

551958LV00001B/10/P